THE PRACTITIONER'S GUIDE TO REFLEXOLOGY

Kevin and
Barbara Kunz

A SPECTRUM BOOK

PRENTICE-HALL, Inc.
Englewood Cliffs, New Jersey 07632

Library of Congress Cataloging-in-Publication Data

Kunz, Kevin.
  The practitioner's guide to reflexology.

  "A Spectrum Book."
  Includes index.
    1. Reflexotherapy.   I. Kunz, Barbara.   II. Title.
[DNLM: 1. Reflexotherapy.   WB 962 K96p]
RM723.R43K867 1985   615.8'2   85-19306
ISBN 0-13-694324-1
ISBN 0-13-694316-0 (pbk.)

10 9 8 7 6 5 4 3 2 1

ISBN 0-13-694324-1

ISBN 0-13-694316-0 {PBK.}

Illustrations by Barbara Kunz
Graphic Art and Design by Betty Colvin
Jacket design by Hal Siegel

*The information in this book is not intended as a substitute for medical
care. If you have a health problem, consult a medical professional.*

This book is available at a special discount when ordered in
bulk quantities. Contact Prentice-Hall, Inc., General
Publishing Division, Special Sales, Englewood Cliffs, N.J. 07632.

Prentice-Hall International (UK) Limited, *London*
Prentice-Hall of Australia Pty. Limited, *Sydney*
Prentice-Hall Canada Inc., *Toronto*
Prentice-Hall Hispanoamericana, S.A., *Mexico*
Prentice-Hall of India Private Limited, *New Delhi*
Prentice-Hall of Japan, Inc., *Tokyo*
Prentice-Hall of Southeast Asia Pte. Ltd., *Singapore*
Whitehall Books Limited, *Wellington, New Zealand*
Editora Prentice-Hall do Brasil Ltda., *Rio de Janeiro*

TABLE OF CONTENTS

1 A THEORY IN MOTION _____ 1
   Why the Feet? _____ 2
   Consider the Foot _____ 6
   The Foot as a Resource _____ 13

2 TECHNIQUE _____ 23
   Stride Replication® Technique _____ 25
   Propriocise® Technique _____ 42

3 THE WORKOUT _____ 53
   The Workouts _____ 67
      Five-Minute Foot Loosener _____ 68
      The Complete Workout _____ 71
      Stride Replication® Workout _____ 78
      Propriocise® Workout _____ 81
   The Workout Workbook _____ 85

4 SPECIAL INTERESTS _____ 105
   Special Interests: Stride Replication® ____ 106
   Special Interests: Propriocise® _____ 122

5 YOU, THE PRACTITIONER _____ 129
   Image of a Profession _____ 130
   Practices of a Profession _____ 131
   The Future of a Profession _____ 134

Postscript _____ 139

Appendix _____ 141

Charts _____ 149

Bibliography _____ 151

Index _____ 153

To Ed Case, Larry Clemmons, Robert Dallamore,
Jill Schneider, and Kenneth Shoemaker

Our thanks to our production crew:
Betty Colvin, Jan and Rol Schneider, Betsy Torjussen,
and Rita Zulka. Our special thanks to the practitioner;
Virginia Anderson, D.R. Blaylock, Mary and Bill Bramlett,
Ellen Case, Vi Coalson, Evelyn Cline, Richard and Joyce
Condon, Darlene Frey, Ruth Hahn, Velma Hein, Jane
Hendricks, Libby Herson, Jim and Sally Ingram, Chris Issel,
Kaora Kanda, Ed Kaufman, Shirley Lyle, Don Mathias, Sara
McCarty, May and Wesley Post, Thelma Rabold, Ken
Renneberg, Twyllah Schauer, Chris Shirley, Jay Skiles,
Margarete Teuwen, Judy Turner, Toni Wilbanks, and many
others. Further thanks to friends of reflexology: Barbara Gale,
Carl Ginsberg, and Clinton Miller.

Other publications by Kevin and Barbara Kunz:
The Complete Guide to Foot Reflexology,
Hand and Foot Reflexology, A Self-Help Guide,
Hand Reflexology Workbook

INTRODUCTION

The practice of reflexology is rich in verbal tradition and a community of believers. Our concern for the last five years has been to bring the practice of reflexology from an informal belief system to a formal profession.

The theory, techniques, and perceptions of a profession presented in this book were gleaned over a five year period of work on feet, literature research, interaction with other reflexologists, and consideration of the role of reflexology. Five years ago we felt the need to find a physiological basis for reflexology to confirm our belief. Four years ago we found that piece of the puzzle through work on feet and literature research. Three years ago the arrest and conviction of a reflexologist prompted us to research a viable role for professional reflexology within society.

As events unfolded over the years, a cohesive body of information emerged. We have labeled this information the Kunz Method of Reflexology. With the publication of *The Practitioner's Guide to Reflexology, The Complete Guide to Foot Reflexology, Hand and Foot Reflexology, A Self-Help Guide,* and *Hand Reflexology Workbook,* we have detailed our observations and study of reflexology.

Shortly before the publication of this book, the Kunz Method of Reflexology was accepted as a form of complementary medicine in England (See Postscript, p. 140). This formal recognition of a practice of reflexology was based on the precepts presented in this book. This information created for us a whole new world of ideas and potential. It is our hope that you will enjoy your exploration.

A Theory in Motion

From the Fiji Islands to Ft. Wayne, Indiana, in present times and from the Pharaohs to the Shogun warriors in ancient times, people have worked on feet. Why the feet? Why have the feet drawn the focused interest of so many for so long? Furthermore, is there a valid premise at the basis of traditional foot work and reflexology, today's representative?

Feet have, indeed, carried man throughout history. Whether climbing a mountain, plowing a field, or standing on a ship's deck, the foot adapts to our chosen terrain. It's a demanding job — an orchestrated balancing act on two pedestals — accomplished through the perception of pressure, stretch, and movement by the feet. Actually, the demands of walking and the role played by pressure, stretch, and movement link us to history, give us a valid definition of reflexology, and point to innovations for the future.

It is our contention that it is the elements of locomotion, pressure, stretch and movement, and the foot's role in perceiving them that have been the real object of foot work throughout the years. In this book, we discuss this physiological basis of reflexology, as well as techniques that replicate pressure, stretch, and movement. Furthermore, we present these sensations to provide definition for reflexology and to identify the role played by the practitioner. Our point of view is taken to define the practice of reflexology within profesional boundaries new to a traditional folk belief system.

WHY THE FEET?

"Do not let it be painful." This interchange between client and practitioner is hauntingly familiar. It accompanies an Egyptian pictograph dating from 2500**B.C.**, yet the conversation could have taken place today as well. What else did ancient man think about in his or her work on feet? The answers to this question are in the artifacts of history.

The pictograph and accompanying hieroglyphs are brief messages. Their placement by the Papyrus Institute of Cairo on exhibit with five other medical practices of ancient times, including dentistry and surgery, provides further information about the role of foot work in this culture. Foot work evidently was linked to health.

Ancient Buddha footsteps in India and Japan indicate a foot-organ relationship reminiscent of today's reflexology theory. A German wood carving dating from the 1500s depicts that culture's attention to the feet, a soaking technique whose use continues today as a unique aspect of

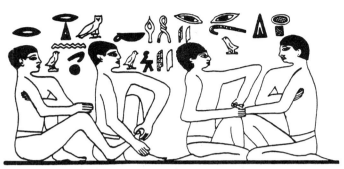

Pictograph and hieroglyphs of work on hands and feet dating from 2500 B.C. in Egypt. (Logo of the Foot Reflexology Awareness Association.)

German reflexology. The discovery and use of foot work in the United States began with the work of Dr. William Fitzgerald in the early 1900s almost simultaneously with the development of a system by a Dr. Hirata in Japan.

The concept of working on feet has been rediscovered over and over again in many different times, in many different cultures. Carl Jung, an eminent Swiss psychologist and psychiatrist, called such phenomena archetypes. *Archetypes* are "Symbolic image(s)... without known origin; and they reproduce themselves in any time or in any part of the world..." (Carl J. Jung, *Man and His Symbols*, Dell Publishing Co., 1968, p.58.) An example of an archetype is shoes and the need to cover one's feet. Virtually every society has found it necessary to consider foot coverage. A further example of an archetype is dentistry and the need to care for teeth.

Imagine the surprise of Ed and Ellen Case when they discovered what is perhaps foot work's most interesting artifact at Cairo's Papyrus Institute. There, hanging in the entryway as one of six medical pictographs, was a pictograph of figures working on hands and feet, dating from approximately 2500 B.C. The hieroglyphs read "Do not let it be painful," and "I do as you please."

Foot work continues today in Germany as a profession allied to the medical profession. A listing of reflexologists is available at pharmacies.

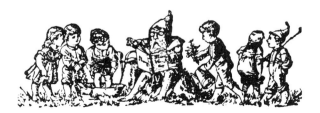

Woodcut of foot-soaking technique dating from the 1500s in Germany. (Contributed by Margarete Teuwen.)

One further attribute of an archetype is spontaneous development, ". . . they reproduce themselves . . . even where transmission by direct descent or 'cross fertilization' through migration must be ruled out." (Carl J. Jung, *Man and His Symbols*, p. 58.) That is to say, the concept of work on feet shows signs of reappearing, rather than being passed on from one culture to another. We have observed this effect in "the naturals," individuals who have never heard of the formalized study of foot work, yet they work on feet purposefully.

Why the feet? What possible linking concepts could exist between these various societies at various times in history? A possible clue lies in the further development of the concept of archetype into archestructure. "An archestructure can now be defined as a felt or perceived function or structural feature of the nervous system, projected or unconsciously

The zones of reflexology and the meridians of acupuncture — are they distant relatives or close cousins? How closely was one modeled after the other? Both use systems of longitudinal body divisors, with the concept that action on one part of the body influences another. Whatever the influence, could both systems have basis in the needs of walking and the whole-body function of locomotion?

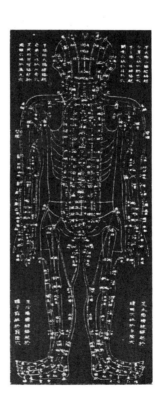

Meridians of acupuncture dating from perhaps 2600 B.C. in China.

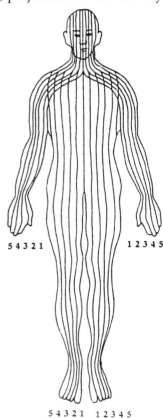

54321   12345

54321   12345

Zones of reflexology dating from early 1900s in the United States.

acted out in the life-style or the beliefs, customs and social structures of the individuals concerned or of whole communities." (Stan Gooch, *Total Man*, Ballantine Books, 1972, p. 299.)

From this interpretation, the pictographs exhibit practices developed to meet a need. Dentistry, for example, is a response to a perceived need, a tooth ache. The dentist has left an archeological and historical trail of the tools of his or her trade. The foot worker has fewer artifacts to leave behind. Historically, the tools of a trade speak of its practice. It is small wonder that foot work leaves a verbal tradition and little physical evidence.

Verbal tradition is a strong part of reflexology today. Word of mouth is the means of communication for instruction and the dissemination of the practice. Does foot work appear throughout history when there is a perceived need for its practice? Is the perceived need acted out unconsciously in the belief in and practice of reflexology?

It may not be clear why ancient man worked on feet or why the naturals work on feet. Today's reflexologist, however, has indicated his or her reasons in a poll conducted by Jill Schneider. (See Appendix.) Furthermore, reflexology has a well-defined belief system fueled by personal observation of its results. In the poll, 100 percent of those answering the poll felt that areas on the feet correspond to the body. The respondents represent thirty-two states of the United States and eleven foreign countries, yet there is a strong commonality of belief represented in their answers.

The practice of foot work in such a variety of cultures throughout history speaks of a universal bridging concept. What could link such diverse groups? And, could such a linkage be defined within the workings of the body's nervous system?

CONSIDER THE FOOT

To be able to move, the body must "see" itself. Such perception requires information about muscles, tendons, and joints. From such information, the body creates a picture of itself. The messengers of self-perception are those that apprise the body of pressure, stretch, and movement — the proprioceptors. Proprioception means, Literally, to perceive oneself. The body makes decisions on the basis of this and other information. The decisions are about how to best allocate resources and, furthermore, how to learn from the experience.

Movement requires the gathering of information, the comparison of this information to past experience, and the determining of the next move. Once a course of action has been decided, instructions about the next step are relayed. Information is again gathered and acted upon. From the incoming messages, the body learns about the success of its intended actions and files this information for further reference.

As the body makes decisions about movement, it also makes decisions in a similar manner about how to fuel the movement. Information is gathered, compared, decided upon, and acted on. Decisions about fuel and movement are made with respect to each. Through the complexity of this activity, the foot is linked to the internal organs. A picture emerges of a possible model for the workings of reflexology within the role of the foot.

The Foot as a Sensory Organ

In order to move, a locomotive apparatus is necessary. As part of the locomotive apparatus, the foot has a sensory function that is not generally recognized. The sensory role of the foot is needed for upright walking, and running should circumstances dictate. The foot senses the ground underfoot.

As with any sensory organ, the foot receives information through sensory experience. The eye, for example, is a sensory organ that processes light as bits of information

**The surface underfoot
signals its characteristics.**

necessary for vision. The foot as a sensory organ processes stretch and pressure as bits of information necessary for locomotion. A movement is made possible by organized packets of information from the sensory organs. The foot, too, gathers packets of information that are necessary for an integrated activity. This is no trivial task. It can be accomplished with ease only by the contraction and relaxation of specific muscle groups throughout the body. To make locomotion possible, these muscle groups respond in sequence. The sequences are signaled by a particular sensory event: the pressure of the surface being walked on, the perceived angle of the terrain, the stretch of the muscle in response to the surface, and the speed at which the surface is encountered. Proprioception — or the perception of pressure, stretch, and movement — is the sensory role of the foot.

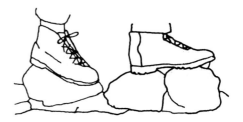

The Role of the Foot in Stride

What are the functions of the foot? This complex system of muscles, ligaments, tendons, and joints supplied by the nervous and circulatory system has two main jobs to perform. The feet provide an upright, stable pedestal to support the body in a stationary position. And the feet provide the leverage necessary to propel us forward in the act of locomotion, or walking. This act requires a structure that is flexible and has the capacity for absorbing shock loads and dispersing them evenly throughout the body.

Muscles contract and relax. It is a cycle. When a muscle needs to perform a function such as lifting the forearm, a set of muscles contracts. When the desired action is over, the muscle relaxes, causing the arm to fall. If it were not for the oppositional muscles, there would be only a one-directional control over a body part. But muscles move in contrast to each other, enabling the arm to lift and to lower. As one muscle contracts, the other relaxes, in an intricate interplay of movement.

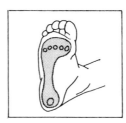

Pressure sensors on a foot during standing.

Anyone who has watched an infant grow can appreciate the complexity of learning body positioning, especially in sitting, standing, and walking. The waving of hands and feet in the newborn exhibits the beginning of a positioning awareness. The intricacies of sitting up are such that it takes two months for the infant to master it. Standing usually requires six months of experimentation and walking takes nine months. The experimentation with possibilities of positions and movements can be seen throughout childhood. Tricycle and bicycle riding are ventures into balancing. Swinging on playground equipment, jumping rope, and other forms of what is considered "play" are actually an educational process for the body. The awkward teenager is living testimony to the fact that this educational process is at least sixteen to eighteen years in duration.

What does this mean in terms of the function of the foot? It makes it possible to maintain posture. A soldier standing at attention is constantly teetering, imperceptibly, back and forth. As he sways forward, the muscles in the back of the leg tighten. As he sways back, the muscles toward the front of the leg tighten to correct the posture. This proprioceptive information is quickly sent and interpreted by the brain to keep the soldier from falling on his face.

What does this mean to the walking mechanism? Sets of oppositional muscles throughout the foot, leg, and hip interplay to tighten certain muscles when needed and to relax others. The effect of these oscillations is a highly skilled, unconscious "pre-set" program of walking. A pre-set program is one that is not consciously thought out each time it is required for use but rather is called up by the brain when needed. What is contained within this program are the cycles of contraction and relaxation performed by the various groups of muscles involved in locomotion throughout the body.

A basketball player, for example, practices to change conscious actions in unconscious movement. These pre-set programs are constantly being reinforced after each attempt. The feedback the player receives helps him to subtly readjust with each shot. The player will vary his practice to allow the body to experience greater flexibility in where and how he shoots. A lay-up shot, although using similar principles, is obviously not the same as a free throw.

The Role of the Foot in Locomotion

The contact the foot initially makes with the ground is called a heel strike. This pressure indicates to the muscles used in this phase of the stride mechanism that it is time to use their specific roles in the stride. The foot rolls forward along the outside edge of the longitudinal arch and then to the metatarsals which form the ball of the foot. Pressure here signifies another segment of the stride mechanism and, thus, triggers another set of specific muscles. The push-off for forward propulsion begins here and ends with the final thrust of the big toe. This "rocking-horse" motion is normally smooth and sliding, with uninterrupted motion from each part of the foot.

The flexibility needed to carry out the stride mechanism efficiently is determined by the sensory demands made on the feet and the on-going educational process provided by these demands. Any interruption in the efficiency of the stride mechanism takes energy from another of the body's functions.

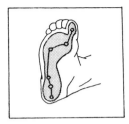

Pressure sensors on a foot during stride.

The Foot as Part of Our Survival Mechanism

In case of danger, the feet participate in the overall body reaction to ensure the survival of the being. This reaction is familiarly known as "fight or flight" because the body gears its internal structures to provide the fuel necessary for either eventuality. The sudden adrenal surge that enables a person to lift a car is an example of this internal reaction. Muscles ready for action are also part of this overall body reaction. The tone of the flexor muscles is increased. Putting up the fists to fight or raising the hands above the head to surrender are both responses to this survival mechanism. The muscles of the feet are a part of the system ready to fight or flee. The feet, too, must be ready to do their part to ensure survival.

The Foot as an Educable Structure

During childhood the foot, along with the rest of the body, receives an education. An exploration of the body's potential and its interaction with other forms of what is considered "play" are actually educational processes for the body. The body's education does not end in childhood, however. Because of the lifelong need to adapt to the constantly changing environment, the body requires lifelong continuing education in the form of sensory information.

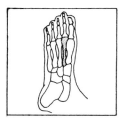

The astronaut and the ballet dancer have one thing in common: the restructuring of bone due to the use of his or her body in these professions. The astronaut actually *loses* bone mass during a space flight. The ballet dancer *gains* bone mass throughout a dancing career.

The common element is Wolff's Law. It states simply that bone will change in external contour and internal architecture according to the intensity and direction of the stresses to which they are habitually subjected. A ballet dancer executes the toe point with a locking wedge of foot bones, with the weight of the body born primarily by the second metatarsal. Due to the habitual use of the bone in this manner, the second metatarsal thickens. In contrast, the astronaut will actually lose bone mass in the heel in response to the relative inactivity of space flight. Because of his weightlessness in space, the astronaut floats rather than walks. No demand is put on the calcaneum, and bone mass is lost.

For those of us in less exotic professions, Wolff's Law still applies. The average woman, for example, loses 30 percent of her total bone mass between the ages of 30 and 70. It is theorized that this is the result of a change in life style during these years. Bedridden patients lose bone mass from the entire skeletal system but particularly from the heel. This takes place within the first two weeks of confinement and becomes significant within fourteen weeks.

It is thus a curious phenomenon that the body will actually change in structure in response to the demands made upon it.

The Role of the Foot in Endorphin Release

The response of the body to pain is an attempt to inhibit it through the release of endorphins, the body's natural pain relievers. The foot participates in this process with every step. To bear the weight of the body in relation to the surface, pain must be managed by the foot. The foot, after all, receives two-and-a-half times the body weight as it acts as a de-accelerator, slowing the body to meet the surface. Endorphins are an insulator in this shock absorption task, insulating the body from too much demand. The demand of pressure, as well as the demand created by acupuncture needles, has been linked to endorphin release.

Are endorphins keyed to the feet in particular? A standard definition of proprioception notes "deep pressure from the bottom of the foot" as one of the sensations that apprises the body of position. Does the foot's role in pressure-sensing key it to endorphin release? Endorphin studies of runners attribute the "runners high" experienced after running to the release of endorphins triggered by the pounding of feet on surface.

Pressure and Pain

"To calm a horse, veterinarians still rely on a device dating back at least to the Middle Ages. It's called the twitch. When this loop of metal or rope is tightened around a horse's upper lip, the animal typically becomes quiet, sometimes even droopy, and meekly submits to a medical treatment or a new set of shoes. Veterinarians have assumed that the pain in the lip merely diverts the horse from reacting to other irritations. Now Dutch scientists have another explanation: The twitch is a Western example of acupuncture....

"An analysis of the horses' blood showed that the twitch nearly doubled the level of endorphins — the natural pain-killers that affect the central nervous system much like morphine. And when the horses were given a drug that blocks the effects of morphine, the twitch no longer sedated the animals. This is the same pattern found in studies of acupuncture. The Dutch researchers conclude that the twitch, like an acupuncture needle, seems to anesthetize by stimulating certain nerve endings to activate the body's pain-killing chemicals...."
"It's Nature's Way of Saying, Whoa," Science 84, Dec. 1984, Vol. 5, No. 10, p.6.

The Foot as a Reflection of the Body

Reiteration is the body's systematic organizational scheme that establishes and maintains a communication throughout the body and thus ensures survival in a potentially hostile environment. The perception and location of a pin prick on the body's surface, for example, is possible because the specialized neuron in a particular location reports to its appropriate area of the brain. Stimulation of the specialized neuron informs the brain of the type of sensation (pain, in this instance). It is of vital importance that the location of the intrusion also be communicated to the brain. A poke in the eye is different from a pat on the back. This is accomplished by the direct link between the body surface and its representative area in the somatic-sensory cortex of the brain. An image of what is taking place, and where, is

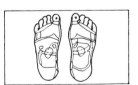

"In man, the nerve segments, which together form the neck and arms, are also the ones where the heart appears. The result is that the nerves bringing sensations from the heart are in the same segment as the nerves which bring sensation from the neck and arm. This relationship is preserved despite the fact that in the course of foetal development the heart migrates to a position which is quite remote from its original site . . . But the heart maintains its ancient Parliamentary representation, despite its position in the body: The neck, arm, and upper chest continue to feel the pain for it. The same form of representation applies to all those parts which one would loosely call the 'innards.' "
Jonathan Miller, *The Body in Question*, Random House, 1978, pp. 23-26.

constructed by reports of sensation to particular parts of the brain. The development of this system begins at conception. The exact process by which a developing neuron finds its way to its appropriate location is unknown.

It is known that certain body systems are linked to others through development. A pain in the arm and shoulder, for example, is a recognized symptom of heart attack because the heart itself does not sense pain, but alarm is sounded by a pre-natal neighbor. The feet may develop a linkage to the body in a similar manner. Similar referred relationships may be present. Rather than a referral of pain, it may be a referral of information necessary for movement or some other purpose. Just as the optic nerves develop a specialty and organize for a special function — sight — there is a concentration in the feet of nerve cells specialized for movement. Why should these cells not organize with attributes of both a referral system and a specialized sensory organ appropriate for the function of movement? Such an organization would require communication of all body parts to allow for the complexity of movement.

In Conclusion

The foot is thus a part of an organized communication system necessary for walking. The information gathered by the foot becomes a part of the body's decision-making process for the allocation of resources. Is it the foot's functions that make it a resourceful part of the body? That is to say, is it the foot's role in walking that provides a link among foot workers?

THE FOOT AS A RESOURCE

The foot communicates with the entire body through the act of locomotion and the language of pressure, stretch, and movement. Pressure, stretch, and movement applied in a consistent program are the tools for working with the foot as a resource to counter stress, save energy, and develop body awareness. The techniques of reflexology, stride replication® , and propriocise® place controlled demands in the body's own language on areas targeted for their role in locomotion. The application of these sensations without the strain of weight bearing and in a consistent manner create an interruption of stress and an internal review for the body.

Model of a Body Under Stress

Walking is a stress, a demand placed on the body to which the body must respond. Hans Selye, stress researcher, describes the adaptation to stress as a three-stage General Adaptive Syndrome. These stages are analagous to the ages of life.

GENERAL ADAPTIVE SYNDROME (Selye)

Adaptive Stage		Ages of Life
Alarm:	"The body shows the changes characteristic of the first exposure to a stressor. At the same time, its resistance is diminished and, if the stressor is sufficiently strong (severe burns, extremes of temperature), death may result."	Childhood
Resistance:	"Resistance ensues if continued exposure to the stressor is compatible with adaptation. The bodily signs characteristic of the alarm reaction have virtually disappeared, and resistance rises above normal."	Adulthood
Exhaustion:	"Following long-continued exposure to the same stressor, to which the body had become adjusted, eventually adaptation energy is exhausted. The signs of the alarm reaction reappear, but now they are irreversible, and the individual dies."	Old Age
	Selye, Hans, *Stress Without Distress*, New American Library, 1974, p. 27.	

A stressor in itself is neither good nor bad from Selye's viewpoint. It is the duration of the stress that is the real wear-and-tear factor. Furthermore, the body has finite energy resources with which to resist a stressor. Selye illustrates this point with an analogy of falling into an icy lake: the initial alarm, the adaptation and resistance, and exhaustion if the stress is not interrupted.

Being pulled from the water interrupts the stressor. While such extreme fight or flight reactions are seldom called for in everyday life, interruption of everyday stressors is acknowledged by weekends, vacations, and holidays. An interruption of stress is a break in routine.

Stress is the process of meeting the world around us. Adapting to demands made upon us is an on-going process. Like any process, it is an improvable skill. The ability to best adapt to stress is a matter of knowing what to request. It is possible to make a request for the best possible adaptation under the circumstances. A request to interrupt the pattern of stress provides a break in the routine, resolving the wear-and-tear aspect of continuous stress.

THE STRESS OF A FOOTSTEP

During a footstep, the body's weight is transferred from heel to toe along a stride path on the sole of the foot. (See illustration of a footstep.) As the foot makes contact with the terrain, chains of muscles throughout the body are keyed to sensors along the stride path. The heel striking the floor, for example, provides information about a portion of the stride path, communicating with the entire body about the foot in relation to the body. The stride path is thus a target area for the application of pressure, stretch, and movement techniques.

The action of a foot during a footstep is to de-accelerate/accelerate and to pitch/roll. This is accomplished as sensors along the stride path signal the appropriate action to take place.

A FOOTSTEP

Footstep Stage	Foot Direction	Role

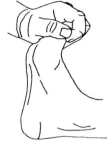

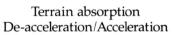

Terrain absorption
De-acceleration/Acceleration

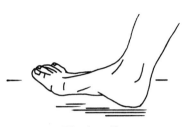

Heel strike

Dorsiflexion

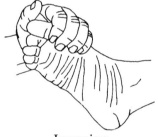

Inversion

Terrain seeking
Pitch

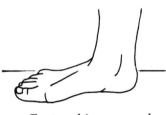

Foot seeking ground

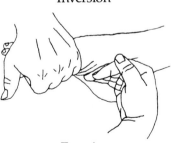

Eversion

Terrain seeking
Roll

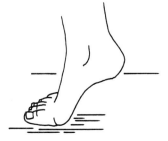

Toe-off

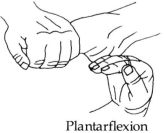

Plantarflexion

Terrain absorption
Acceleration

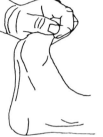
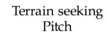

INTERRUPTING THE STRESS OF WALKING

Shoes and flat surfaces add to the stress of walking. Adulthood and civilization thus join to create a lessened sensory demand on the feet and the body as a whole. The foot as a sensory organ that detects terrain and adapts to it is no longer given the opportunity to practice its full capabilities. The foot as a functional part of locomotion over-uses certain capabilities and under-uses others.

Reflexology, stride replication®, and propriocise® techniques provide a variety of sensory experience and demand which interrupts the pattern of stress created by walking. The techniques as applied by the practitioner are requests in the body's own language, using the foot as a terminal to ask the body to interrupt its present programming and pay attention to the request. The request is one for change, an interruption in stress.

The application of pressure, stretch, and movement techniques create an alarm situation in Selye terms, a demand to which the body must respond. The adaptation to this input is a form of learning. As in any learning situation, the consistency and frequency of practice play a role in the learning process. By thus choosing such stressors, it is possible to interact with the exhaustion phase of Selye's stress model. Through the practice of the foot's full capabilities, stress is interrupted and the body learns. As a long-term result, the body is given practice at information-gathering and making best possible adaptation on the basis of the fuller information. Choose it and use it are at the core of this learning process.

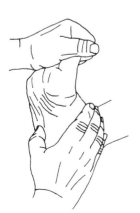

Reflexology technique

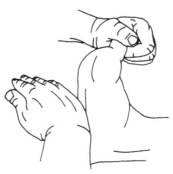

Stride replication® technique

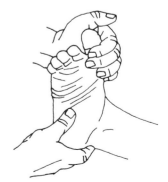

Propriocise® technique

Application of Technique

Choosing the program of pressure, stretch, and movement which is used takes into consideration the role of the foot in locomotion. The techniques of reflexology, stride replication®, and propriocise® offer the exercise of the foot's full capabilities. Each technique series has as its goal the practice of a primary sensory signal.

PRIMARY SENSORY SIGNALS

Technique Series	Signals of Pressure	Signals of Stretch	Signals of Movement
Reflexology	primary	some	some
Stride Replication®	some	primary	some
Propriocise®	some	some	primary

Application of technique is based on the principles of body relationship associated with the technique series. The relationship is established by the body's response to locomotive demands. The techniques of reflexology are a response to the demands of alignment with gravity, coordination of all body parts during movement, and pressure sensing by the foot. For further information about the properties of technique application see "The Workout Workbook," p. 85 . (See also Kunz and Kunz, *The Complete Guide to Foot Reflexology*, Prentice-Hall, Inc., 1982, and *Hand Reflexology Workbook*, Prentice-Hall, Inc., 1985.)

STRIDE REPLICATION® TECHNIQUE

Stride replication® techniques recognize the demands of changing terrain. The angle at which the foot hits the ground during a footstep and the path along which the foot makes contact with the ground are the locomotive demands recreated by stride replication® techniques.

In a footstep the foot is placed in position to meet the ground by the interaction of four major muscle groups. The stretch of these major muscle groups becomes the object for the application of stride replication® technique, in addition to the sole of the foot, which is targeted for its pressure-sensing capabilities.

Moving Through a Footstep

The foot has the ability to move in many directions and to be placed in many positions. Almost all are the result of a combination of muscles which make possible the movement of the foot in four basic directions. (Note the position of the sole of the foot in the illustrations. The four basic directional movements of the foot result in the placement of the sole of the foot in relation to the body, as shown.)

Actually, each of the basic foot directions plays a role in moving the foot through the stage of a footstep. The foot must be in the proper position as it strikes the ground or the many muscles throughout the body involved in stride are unable to efficiently and effectively fulfill their roles. The effect is similar to uneven wear of tires on a car whose wheels are out of alignment.

A quadrant system for technique application is established by recognition of the muscle group most responsible for moving the foot in a basic direction. (See chart.)

Quadrant System
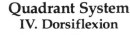
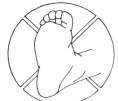

IV. Dorsiflexion

III. Eversion   **I. Inversion**

II. Plantarflexion

In the body's language, the need for the foot to move in a basic direction is signaled by the perception of pressure to the bottom of the foot during a footstep. Chains of muscles throughout the body are keyed to this perception of pressure so that they can play their role in positioning the body itself during a footstep. Pressure to the bottom of the foot, particularly to the stride path, conveys information about the surface being walked on, the perceived angle of the terrain, the stretch of muscle in response to the surface, and the speed at which the surface is encountered.

In stride replication® techniques, the role of the foot in positioning itself and perceiving pressure during stride become a means with which to communicate with the body. Pressure, stretch, and movement techniques are applied to the foot to provide a variety of sensation and, thus,

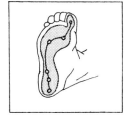

Four Basic Foot Directional Movements

	Direction	Primary muscle group responsible for directional movement

I N V E R S I O N

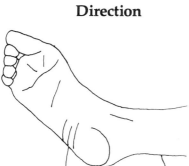

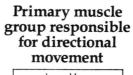
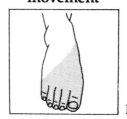

I

P L A N T A R F L E X I O N

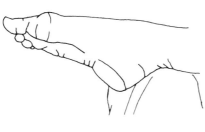

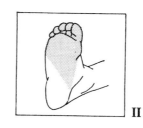

II

E V E R S I O N

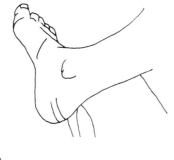

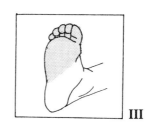

III

D O R S I F L E X I O N

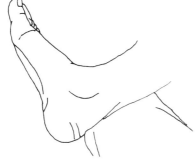

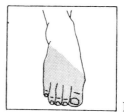

IV

relaxation of over-used and under-used muscles. An exercise of the foot's full capabilities through the relaxation/contraction cycle of muscles is the goal of technique application.

Consider the Foot's Day

Adaptation to shoes and modern surfaces has implications for the foot. Shoes and flat, hard surfaces over-exercise certain parts of the foot and under-exercise other parts. When walking on concrete, for example, the foot over-uses its shock absorbers and under-uses its terrain seekers. Note the foot in each illustration and consider the "exercise" each receives during the course of a day.

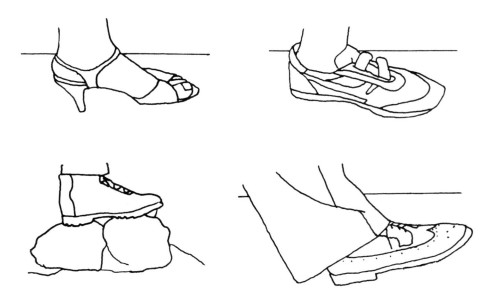

PROPRIOCISE® TECHNIQUE

Propriocise® is the practice and development of body position not normally experienced in everyday life. Flexibility and full range of motion contribute to the body's ability to move about most efficiently. Propriocise® techniques practice movement and integration of basic movements of the foot.

   Propriocise® techniques also exercise the capabilities of the joint and interrupt the routine operating pattern of movement. Focus on the joints by the pressure, stretch, and movement techniques of propriocise® creates a focus for effect on the muscles, tendons, and ligaments related to that joint. Relaxation, flexibility, and, in the long run, less wear and tear are the goals of propriocise® technique application.

The Goals of the Practitioner

Through the application of pressure, stretch, and movement techniques, the goals of the practitioner are:

- the interruption of stress
- prevention of the wear and tear of under-use and over-use
- a method of working with past stressors
- enhancement of body awareness
- energy savings through practice of locomotive elements.

IN CONCLUSION

The inclusion of a foot work system by many cultures throughout history has a potential link in the role of the foot during locomotion. Does foot work represent a type of bipedal maintenance, a needed exercise of the foot's repertoire? We feel that there is ample evidence to support this idea, as well as to stimulate ongoing innovations within the practice of reflexology.

Technique

The techniques of reflexology, stride replication® and propriocise® practice pressure, stretch, and movement to mimic the body's own language of deep pressure to the bottom of the feet, stretch of muscle, angulation of joint, and tempo of action. Reflexology techniques for the practitioner are discussed in other Kunz and Kunz works: *The Complete Guide to Foot Reflexology*, Prentice-Hall, Inc., 1982 and *Hand Reflexology Workbook*, Prentice-Hall, Inc., 1985.

Stride replication® and propriocise® techniques presented in this book complement the traditional pressure techniques of reflexology, adding stretch and movement techniques for a full range of sensory experience to the foot.

Each technique series — stride replication® and propriocise® — has as its goal the application of pressure, stretch, and movement. While the primary sensory signal of each series is different, both share common qualities of technique application.

All techniques are described in terms of two steps: the preparation of technique made by a holding hand and the application of technique made by a working hand. Note in the technique descriptions that the role of the holding hand varies, sometimes equaling the role of the working hand. The goal of the practitioner is to most efficiently and effectively combine the efforts of the holding hand and working hand.

Stride Replication® Technique

The techniques of stride replication® mirror a footstep and the foot's role in terrain absorption and terrain seeking. The gauges of pressure, stretch, and movement make possible a footstep. It is these sensations that provide a means of communication in the body's language.

The mimicry of these sensations provides variety to the foot and makes possible an interruption of the foot's stress pattern. The techniques of stride replication® are a recognition of the body's protective mechanism which quickly relaxes in response to extreme stretch. The techniques place the foot in a position of stretch and a sensory signal is applied. When the foot meets a force or weight of a particular stretch, the foot relaxes to meet the weight rather than incur injury. While the application of stride replication® techniques is not of sufficient force to cause damage, the application is interpreted by the body as a need to relax quickly. Muscle groups throughout the body that also are involved in a footstep relax as well.

In particular, the techniques are applied to parts of the foot that play an important role in stride. The stride path on the sole of the foot and the four major muscle groups that move the foot are the primary targets to which the techniques are applied. Evaluation of the application of the techniques is more fully discussed in "The Workout."

The application of stride replication® techniques is most comfortably applied by considering the positioning of the practitioner, the working hand, and the holding hand. The practitioner sits facing the soles of the feet. Note the position of the working hand and arm in the illustration. The goal

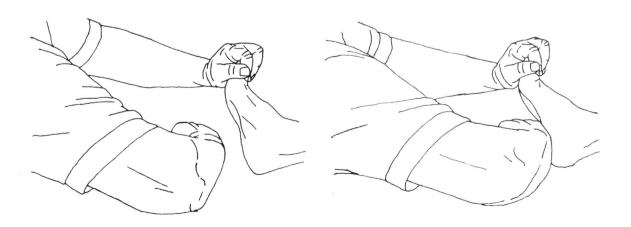

of the technique application is to make contact repeatedly with a surface of the hand and a surface of the foot. The real activity is in the role of the working arm with a bending/unbending at the elbow and/or a movement at the shoulder. The active participation of the working arm in stride replication® techniques calls upon a muscle use different from that of reflexology. One consideration in the application of the techniques is prevention of fatigue. Give yourself time to develop the necessary muscles by gradually increasing the duration of technique application.

The testing of stride replication® techniques is separate from the application of the technique. In reflexology and propriocise® techniques, one feels or tests as one works. The testing of a stride replication® technique or technique series takes place after the technique or techniques are applied. Basically, the ankle is tested by turning the foot in a circle and assessing the resistance to a smooth turn.

Stride replication® techniques are presented in this chapter with an evaluative phase, the circling technique. The evaluative aspects of the circling technique will be more fully presented in "The Workout." In practicing the stride replication® techniques, however, circling adds interest and a transition between technique application.

TESTING: THE CIRCLING TECHNIQUE

Circling is a full 360° turn of the ankle. A full turn is necessary to most closely replicate the ankle's full repertoire of movement. In addition, particular note is taken of the feel of the circling technique as the foot moves through the four quadrants.

Grasp the foot as shown and turn the foot in a circle.

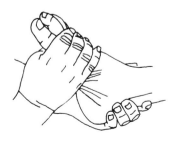

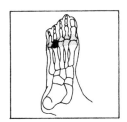

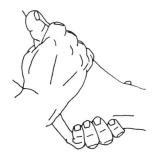
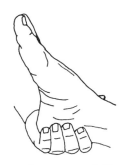

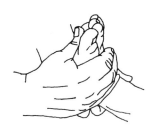

To gain better control over the foot and to turn a fuller circle, consider first the role of the hand that cups the heel — the holding hand. In addition to cupping the heel, the hand pulls on the heel slightly to isolate the movement of the foot.

The working hand grasps the upper foot around the metatarsal heads. The entire palm surface of the hand makes contact with the foot. The flat of the thumb is positioned on the bottom of the foot on the surface covering the fourth metatarsal head. The flats of the index and middle fingers are placed on top of the foot over the fourth metatarsal head.

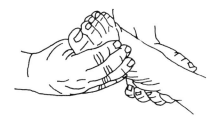

The foot is moved with the guidance of the thumb and fingers on the fourth metatarsal head to trace a circle in the air with the tip of the big toe. To turn the right foot in a full clockwise circle, push with the flat of the thumb as the foot is moved through the circle segment indicated in the illustration. At a certain movement, the flats of the fingers add to the continuation of the circle by the flat of the thumb. The flats of the fingers then move the foot through the next segment of the circle. After another brief moment where both thumb and fingers move the foot, the flat of the thumb pushes and continues the movement of the foot.

After several successive circles, practice a counterclockwise circle. The roles of thumb and fingers are reversed in the previous discussion.

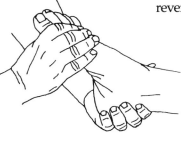

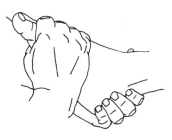

WORKING HAND

In stride replication® techniques, an important role is played by the movement of the working arm. The working arm bends and unbends at the elbow bringing the hand into contact with the foot. A swinging pendulum motion, pivoted at the elbow, establishes a smooth, fluid application and a rhythmic tempo. Also, positioning the working hand and arm in relationship to the foot, the practitioner creates a comfortable working situation.

In summary, the application of stride replication® techniques is made a comfortable experience for both client and practitioner by considering the role played by the working hand and arm.

The goal of the technique is to provide variety of sensory experience and relaxation to the foot.

A point of contact is created in stride replication® techniques by the use of an "edge" of the hand as a working surface. (See illustrations.) Use of the padded edges of the hand as a working surface gives focus to the technique and comfort to the subject. The practitioner works with a defined point of contact to meet a chosen surface of the foot. The point of contact appropriate to each technique is discussed with the technique description.

Care should be taken with the application of techniques. Excessive force in application may cause injury. The top and sides of the foot are thinly muscled and may become reddened if the techniques are applied in an overly vigorous manner. Also, the foot may redden if the techniques are applied as more of a slap than a cup, tap, or percussion.

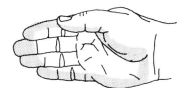

Cupping

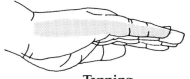

Tapping

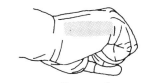

Percussion

Pivot at elbow

Point of contact

Tempo

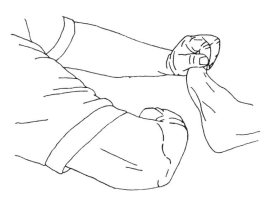

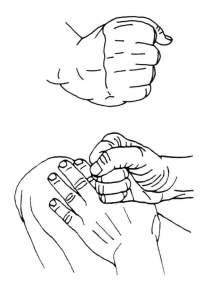

Percussion

Form the hand into a loose fist. The object of the technique is to make contact with the padded outside edge of the hand. The elbow is the only moving part of the working arm. The bicep remains flexed throughout. Draw the right arm toward the chest and swing it forward, making contact with the hand. Set up a rhythm. Don't try to use too much force. Force is not as important as a rapid stretch of the muscle. The tempo, which can be established by the flexing of the bicep throughout the technique, is more important than force.

To practice percussion, rest your hand on your leg. (See illustration.) Apply the technique of percussion.

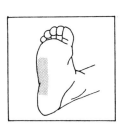
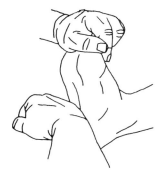

Holding hand (L): Rest the heel of the hand on the ball of the foot. The foot is drawn taut by the control of the toes by the working fingers. **Working hand (R):** Note the intended working surface, as indicated in the illustration. Consider the surface of the working hand that makes contact with the foot in this technique. Apply the percussion technique to the area indicated.

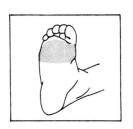
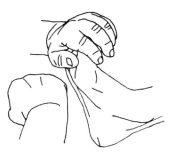

Holding hand (L): Position the hand to accommodate the actions of the working hand on the intended working surface.
Working hand (R): Apply the percussion technique to the working surface. Note that the working hand makes contact across the ball of the foot.

Holding hand (L): Hold the foot comfortably taut.

Working hand (R): Note the position of the working hand. Contact with the foot is made by the usual padded outside edge of the hand.

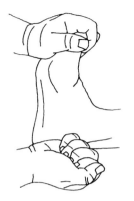 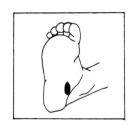

Holding hand (L): Hold the foot comfortably taut.

Working hand (R): On the foot, note the intended working surface. To make technique application a comfortable experience, the lack of padding on this part of the foot is compensated for by use of the padding of the working hand. Tighten the fist to provide increased padding. Apply the percussion technique.

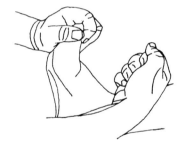 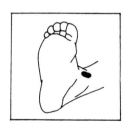

Holding hand (L): Hold the foot comfortably taut.

Working hand (R): Note the position of the working hand. Apply the percussion technique.

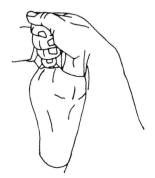 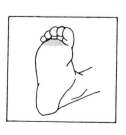

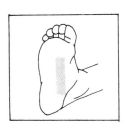

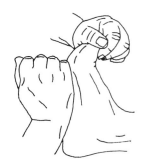

Holding hand (L): Hold the foot comfortably taut.

Working hand (R): Apply the percussion technique. Note that the length of the working hand surface makes contact with the foot.

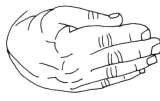

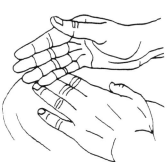

Tapping

In the technique of tapping, the outside of the little finger of an open, relaxed hand makes contact with the foot. The effect is like rapping a closed hand-fan on the knee. The ribs of the fan rap together. In tapping, the fingers of the hand tap together. To achieve this effect, the fingers must be relaxed (not stiff as in a karate chop).

To practice tapping, try this technique on your thigh. Keep the hand open and the fingers relaxed. Can you hear the fingers slap together, making a tap, tap, tapping sound? The goal of tapping is achieved by a rapid, rhythmic stroke, not a forceful blow. Force may cause injury or discomfort.

The movement of the working arm is the same as that used in the technique of percussion. The bicep of the arm is flexed, and the arm is turned so that the outside of the hand can make contact with the foot. Unlike percussion, the hand is open and the contact is made with the outside of the little finger. The elbow is the only moving part of the working arm. The bicep remains flexed throughout.

Heavy Medium Light

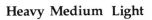

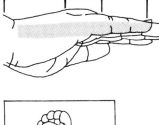

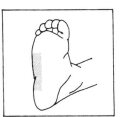

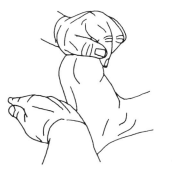

Holding hand (L): Hold the foot comfortably taut.

Working hand (R): Note the intended working surface. Consider the surface of the working hand that makes contact with the foot. In the tapping technique, this surface determines the application of technique as light, medium, or heavy. Apply the tapping technique. Experiment with the light, medium, and heavy working surfaces of the working hand.

Holding hand (L): The holding hand is positioned to accommodate the action of the working hand.
Working hand (R): Apply the tapping technique. Note that the working hand makes contact across the ball of the foot. Experiment with the surface of the working hand that makes contact with the foot.

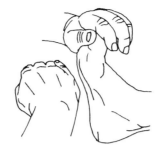 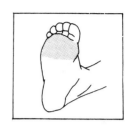

Holding hand (L): Accommodate the working hand. Note that the heel of the holding hand holds the foot taut.
Working hand (R): Apply the tapping technique. Experiment with the light, medium, and heavy working surfaces of the working hand.

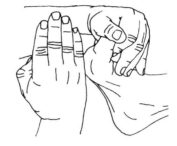 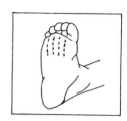

Holding hand (L): Grasp the toes and steady the toe being worked.
Working hand (R): Apply the tapping technique.

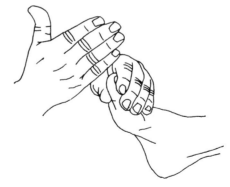 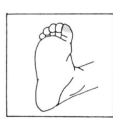

Holding hand (L): Hold the foot comfortably taut.
Working hand (R): Apply the tapping technique. Note that the length of the working hand surface makes contact with the foot.

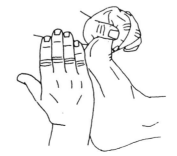 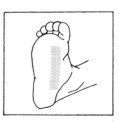

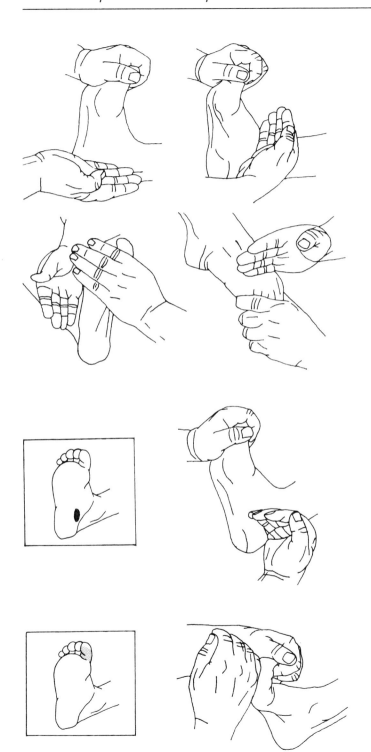

Holding hand (L): Hold the foot comfortably taut.

Working hand (R): Apply the tapping technique. Note that the less padded surfaces of the foot are most comfortably worked with the light working surface of the hand.

Variation:

Curved fingers

Holding hand (L): Hold the foot comfortably taut.

Working hand (R): Hold the hand comfortably, with the fingers slightly curled. Apply the tapping technique. The surface of the working hand is light.

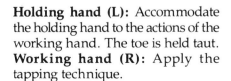

Holding hand (L): Accommodate the holding hand to the actions of the working hand. The toe is held taut.

Working hand (R): Apply the tapping technique.

Cupping

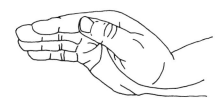

In cupping, the hand pockets air to form a muffled clap. To begin, cup your hand as though scooping water from a stream. To practice the technique, clap the cupped hands together. The sound made should be a dull thud.

Try this technique on the hand. The cup of the hand should be shaped to the surface for maximum effect. This is achieved by varying the curve of the fingers.

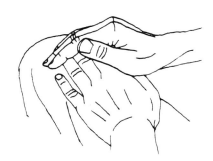

Holding hand (L): Hold the foot comfortably taut.
Working hand (R): On the foot, note the intended working surface. In cupping, the working hand conforms to the surface. In addition to the contact of the "rim" of the cupped hand, the hand conforms to position the heel of the hand to meet the hollows on the foot. Apply the cupping technique.

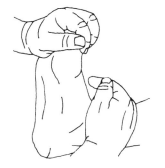 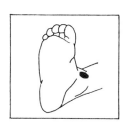

Holding hand (L): Hold the foot comfortably taut.
Working hand (R): Note the changed position of the working arm. It may be necessary to reposition your body to accommodate the arm's work. Apply the cupping technique.

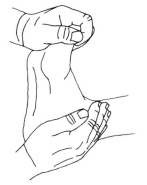 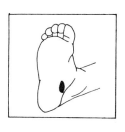

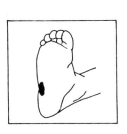
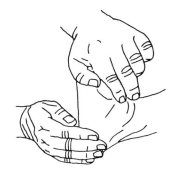

Holding hand (L): Note the changed position of the holding hand to allow the application of the technique to the intended area of the foot. Hold the foot in place.
Working hand (R): Apply the cupping technique. Reposition your body to accommodate the arm's work.

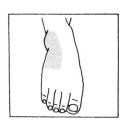
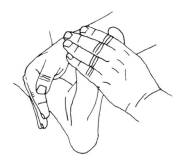

Holding hand (L): The foot is held in position by the holding fingers to accommodate the working hand.
Working hand (R): Note the position of the working hand and consider the position of your body necessary to comfortably apply the technique. Apply the cupping technique.

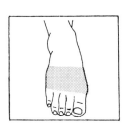
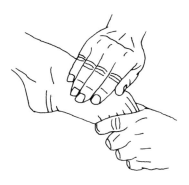

Holding hand (L): Grasp the toes and position the foot.
Working hand (R): Note that the working surface has virtually no muscular padding to absorb the impact of the technique. Exaggerate the cup of the hand when applying the technique to avoid slapping a sensitive part of the foot.

Variation:

Double cupping
Holding and working hands play an
equal role. The foot rests comfortably
on its own. The goal of the technique
is to simultaneously cup the ankle
bones. The rim of the cupped hand
conforms to the surface around the
ankle bone.

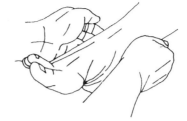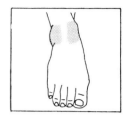

Holding and working hands play an
equal role. Note the position of your
body in relation to the foot. The goal
of the technique is to simultaneously
cup the bottom and top of the foot.
Each cupped hand accommodates a
different working surface.

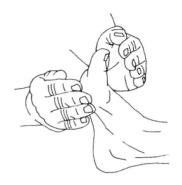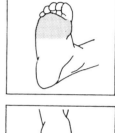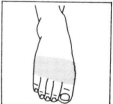

HOLDING HAND

In stride replication® techniques, the holding hand places
the foot in one of four basic positions.

The foot is positioned and held in place by the interplay
of the palm of the hand and the fingers, which act as a unit.
The palm and fingers act in opposition to each other to
create a levering effect and place the foot in a position of
stretch. The foot is held comfortably and efficiently in place.
The focus of the holding hand is control of the foot's own
positioners. For example, the foot in the illustration is held
in place by the control of the toes by the palm of the hand
and fingers. In the technique descriptions, note the role of
the holding hand to control the foot in each of the four basic
positions.

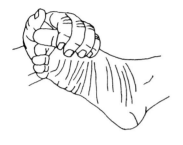

Inversion

Inversion is the turning of the sole of the foot toward the midline of the body. (See illustrations.) To practice the positioning of the foot, grasp the foot as shown. The palmar surface of the hand makes contact with the foot. Control of the foot is achieved by the placement of the heel of the hand on the surface of the foot covering the metatarsal bones and the placement of the fingers in a grasp of the foot. The fingers act as a unit and the entire palmar surface of the hand is involved in movement of the foot. Exert pressure with the heel of the hand. Pull with the fingers. Experiment with the interaction between the palm of the hand and the fingers. Note that the primary action involves the metatarsal heads.

To practice inversion and the application of a technique, apply cupping, tapping, or percussion to the area of the foot, as illustrated.

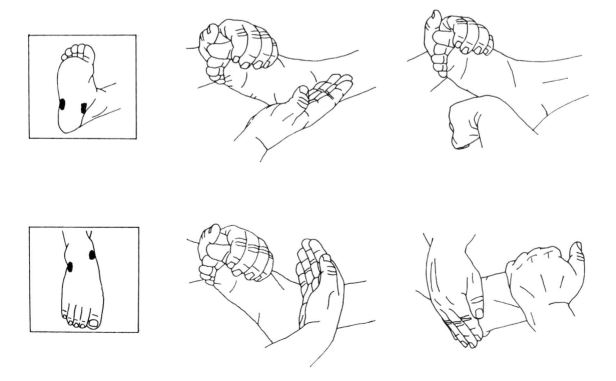

Eversion

Eversion is the turning of the sole of the foot away from the mid-line of the body. To practice this basic position, grasp the foot as shown. Turn the foot away from the mid-line of the body. Note that the primary action is taken on the metatarsal heads by the interplay of the palm of the hand and fingers. Note the actions taken by the holding hand to accommodate the working hand in the illustrations.

To practice eversion and the application of cupping, tapping, and percussion, apply a technique to each of the four basic directional movers of the foot.

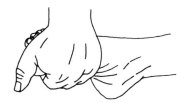

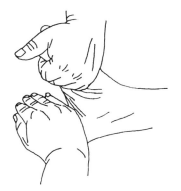
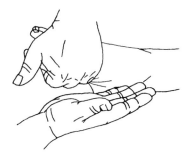
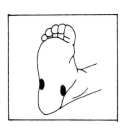

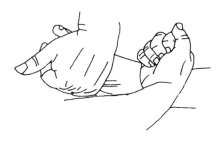
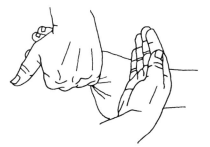
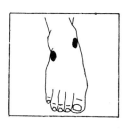

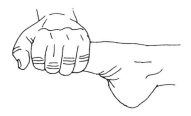

Plantarflexion

Plantarflexion is the positioning of the foot in a toes-pointed position. Control of the foot is in the control of the toes. Grasp the foot as shown. The hand rests on the metatarsal heads and the fingers grasp the toes to maintain the foot's posiiton. Note the actions taken by the holding hand to accommodate the working hand.

To practice plantarflexion and the application of technique, place the foot in position with the holding hand and then with the working hand apply cupping, tapping, or percussion to each of the four basic directional movers of the foot and the top of the foot.

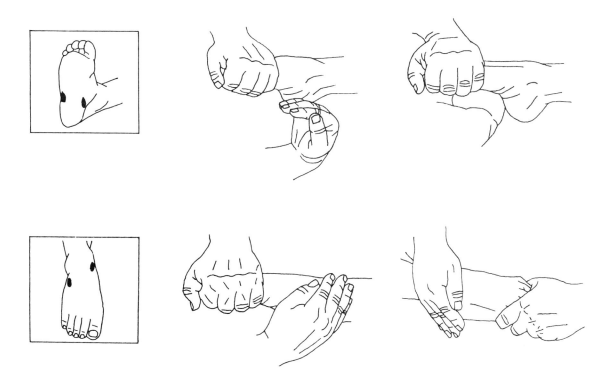

Dorsiflexion

In the *dorsiflexion* position, the sole of the foot faces the practitioner. To practice this positioning, grasp the foot as shown. The heel of the hand rests at the base of the toes and the fingers grasp the toes to control them and the foot's position. Note the actions taken by the holding hand to accommodate the working hand.

To practice dorsiflexion and the application of technique, follow the illustrations.

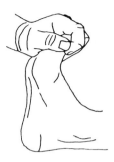

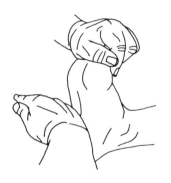

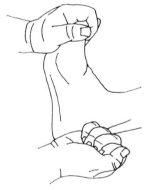

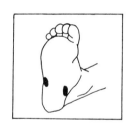

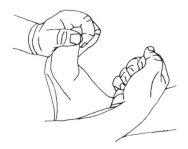

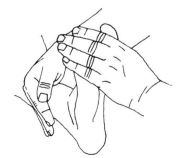

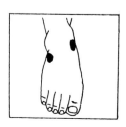

Propriocise® Technique

To perceive oneself, information is gathered from muscles, tendons, and joints. Propriocise® is the practice and development of body position not normally experienced in everyday life. The foot is limited by shoes and surfaces. Propriocise® techniques provide exercise of movements not routinely practiced.

In the learning and practice of propriocise® techniques, care should be taken in their application. No moves are sharp or sudden. If the client reports discomfort at the application of a technique, discontinue use. While it is the goal of the holding and working hands to create leverage with respect to each other, this leveraging ability should not be used to excess. Consider each pair of feet in the application of technique. Smaller, thinner, injured, or older feet call for a gentler approach and may not even be suitable for the application of all techniques. When in doubt, don't do it.

The techniques of propriocise® explore and encourage movement. The goal of the practitioner is to use subtlety in interplay of the holding and working hands with the foot. The movement observations made by the practitioner in the application of technique offer the practitioner a fuller evaluation of the foot.

HOLDING AND WORKING HANDS

In propriocise® techniques, the role of the holding hand is a more active one than the holding hand of reflexology and stride replication® techniques. The holding hand acts to create appropriate conditions and to counter the actions of the working hand. The net result is an enhancement of the movement practiced. In the heel-to-toe mover technique, for example, the holding hand moves the foot in a direction counter to the movement of the working hand. In the foot-flicking technique, the actions of the working hand are enhanced by the role played by the holding hand as it pulls at the ankle and isolates movement of the foot.

In the technique descriptions, note the role played by each hand. Practice the role of each hand separately before combining the work of the two hands. To get the two hands to work together, note the intended movement of the foot and consider it as a goal for the integrated actions of the working and holding hands.

FOOT SCULPTING

The goal of a foot-sculpting technique is to practice the pivoting of the foot. The working hand is sculpted to the foot; that is to say, the entire surface of the hand participates in the movement of the foot even though discrete portions of the hand exert the focused pressure that creates movement. For example, in the metatarsal fan technique as applied to the bottom of the foot, the foot begins the technique in a dorsiflexion position and is then moved alternately into an eversion or inversion position. Thus, foot-sculpting techniques in general offer the practice, or integration, of movement through basic foot direction.

Metatarsal Fan

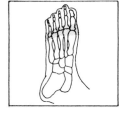

Bottom of the foot
Place the heel of the working hand on the ball of the foot. The fingers grasp the toes to steady the foot. The heel of the hand fans across the metatarsal heads creating movement of the foot. To practice the technique, push with the heel of the hand and roll across the ball of the foot. Move the foot first to the outside and then to the inside. Repeat the pattern of movement several times.

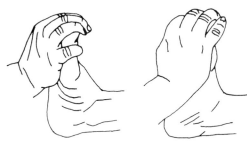

Top of the foot
Place the heel of the hand on top of the foot, as shown. To practice the technique, push with the heel of the hand and roll across the metatarsal heads.

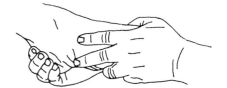

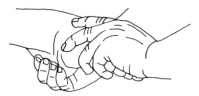

Side to side

The goal of the technique is to emphasize the ability of the upper foot to pivot.

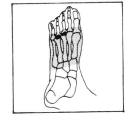

Grasp the foot with the working hand. (Right hand in illustration.) The holding hand grasps the foot to steady it. Position the flat of the working thumb on the bottom surface of the foot over the fourth metatarsal head. Push with the flat of the thumb and move the foot to the outside. Now, move the foot in a counter direction by pushing with the flats of the working fingers on top of the foot. Repeat the pattern of movement several times.

Position the flat of the working thumb on the third metatarsal head and repeat.

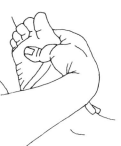

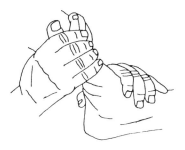

Position the hands as shown. Both hands play an equal role in this technique. The right hand in the illustration and the left hand move counter to each other to create the position of the foot. In the first illustration, the right hand moves the foot toward the subject while the left hand draws the foot away from the subject. In the second illustration, the roles of the right and left hands are reversed. Repeat the pattern of movement. It is possible to achieve a rapid movement of the foot.

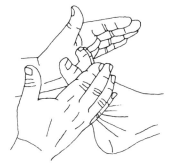

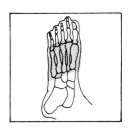

Heel-to-toe mover

The goal of the technique is to move the top portion of the foot, accentuating the movement by the holding and countermovement of the heel of the foot.

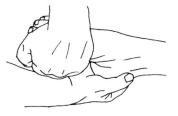

Grasp the foot with the working hand. (Left hand in the illustration.) Cup the heel of the foot in the holding hand. Push with the heel of the working hand and the heel of the holding hand. Note the movement of the foot. Now, to move the foot in a counter direction, pull with the fingers of the working hand and the fingers of the holding hand. Repeat the pattern of movement/countermovement several times.

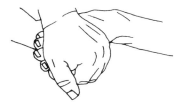

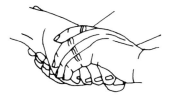

Grasp the foot with the working hand and cup the heel of the foot in the holding hand. Push with the heel of the working hand and pull with the fingers of the holding hand. Note the movement of the foot. Now, to move the foot in a counter direction, pull with the fingers of the working hand and push with the heel of the holding hand. Repeat the pattern of movement/countermovement several times.

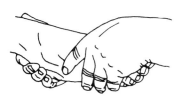

PLANTAR ROCKER

In this technique, the foot is placed in a toes-pointed (plantarflexion) position and rocked gently across the flat of the holding thumb by the actions of the working hand. The goal of this technique is to contrast movement in various parts of the feet. Movement is accentuated by the placement of and pressure exerted by the flat of the thumb of the holding hand.

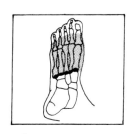

To practice this technique, cup the heel of the foot with the holding hand. (Right hand in the illustration.) The flat of the thumb is placed at the base of the metatarsals, and the fingers act as a unit to provide leverage for the thumb. The working hand grasps the foot. The palm on the hand makes contact with the surface of the foot and acts on the metatarsal heads to move the foot.

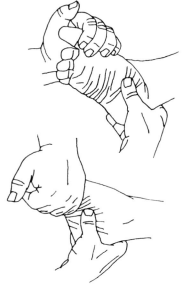

Bring the foot into a toes-pointed position. Rock the palm of the working hand across the top of the foot. The palm is rolled across the foot from the heel of the hand to the base of the fingers. Then to create a countermovement, the palm is rolled across the foot from the base of the fingers to the heel of the hand. The fingers grasp the first metatarsal to accomplish this.

The pattern of movement/countermovement creates a rocking motion as the foot is moved across the flat of the holding thumb.

Care should be taken to apply the technique as a practice of movement. Do not force the foot by exerting extreme pressure. Injury could result.

Go on to the base of the second metatarsal and repeat. Repeat with each metatarsal.

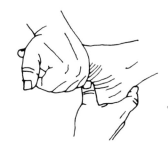

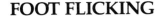

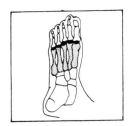

FOOT FLICKING

The goal of foot flicking is to move the foot rapidly in an up-and-down motion. The holding hand grasps the heel to provide a basis of support and to allow the foot to bend at the ankle. The thumb and two fingers of the working hand are placed on the first metatarsal head, with the thumb on the bottom of the foot and the fingers on the top. Each finger is placed slightly to the side of the metatarsal head. (The right hand is used to work the left foot and the left, to work the right foot.) Push up with the thumb to move the foot toward the subject. (See illustration.)

Push down with the two fingers to move the foot toward you. (See illustration.)

Now try this technique moving the foot more quickly in an upward and then downward direction. (See illustration.)

The effect that is achieved is a rapid rhythmic motion of the foot. There is no need to force the foot. The rapidly changing position of the foot is the goal.

In a similar manner, apply the technique to each metatarsal head.

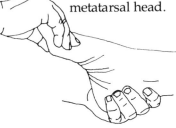

Variation:

Use one finger directly on top of the metatarsal head to move the foot toward you. (See illustration.) Use the thumb on the bottom of the foot to push up on the metatarsal head. (See illustration.) The effect of using one finger on top of the metatarsal head is to fine tune the feeling of vibration created by this technique. This variation may be more appropriate for use on smaller feet.

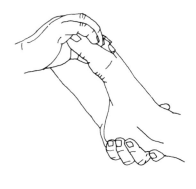

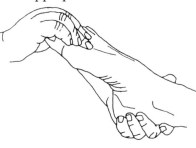

Variation:

With the working hand, grasp the toe. The application of technique is the same as above.

The goal of this technique is relaxation. It may not be appropriate for use with a very stiff ankle. It may even be painful. If so, try other loosening techniques such as cupping, percussion, or tapping.

Care also should be taken to ensure that the fingers of the working hand do not dig into or stretch the potentially sensitive top of the foot.

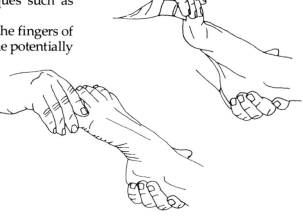

METATARSAL LEVER

The goal of the technique is to work with the metatarsal bones. The working hand (right hand in the illustration) is positioned at the metatarsal head, and the holding hand is positioned at the metatarsal base. The flats of thumb and fingers of both hands are the points of contact with the foot. The holding hand counters the actions of the working hand.

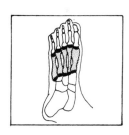

To practice the technique, grasp the foot as shown. Push with the flat of the working thumb and with the flats of the holding fingers. Then, to create countermovement, push with the flats of the working fingers and the flat of the holding thumb. repeat the pattern of movement/counter-movement several times.

Go on to the next metatarsal bone and repeat. Repeat with each metatarsal bone.

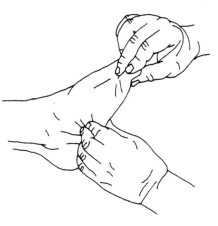

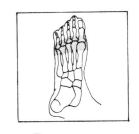

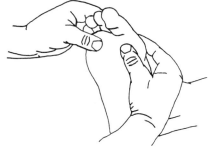

METATARSAL GRASP

The goal of the technique is to create movement between the metatarsal bones. Grasp the foot as shown. Both hands play an equal working role. The flats of thumbs and fingers are the points of contact with the foot. To practice the technique, push with the flat of the right-hand thumb and with the flats of the left-hand fingers. The net result is that the actions of one hand counter the actions to the other hand and thus create an exaggerated foot position. Repeat the pattern of movement/countermovement several times.

Repeat with the other metatarsal bones.

SIDE-TO-SIDE MOVEMENT

The goal of the technique is to practice the slight side-to-side movement of the toes. The working hand creates the movement, while the holding hand counters the movement by serving as a brace.

The working and holding hands grip the tips and joints of the toes. The flats of the thumbs and index fingers of both hands serve as levering points. The goal of the technique is the focused movement of the first joint of the toe by the working hand.

To try the technique, grip the toe as shown. The left hand in the illustration is the working hand. Push with the flat of the working thumb. repeat the movement/counter-movement several times. The holding hand counters this movement with a pull from the index finger. Now move the toe in a counter direction, pushing with the flat of the working index finger against the push of the holding thumb. The movement of the toe is exaggerated by the interplay of the working and holding hands. The toe is rocked between the thumb of one hand and the index finger of the other.

Go on to the next toe and repeat. Repeat with each toe.

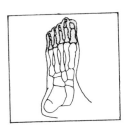

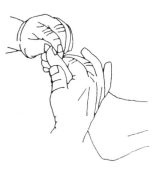

PULL TECHNIQUES

Grasp the toe with the working hand. (Left hand in illustration.) The holding hand grasps the foot with focused pressure at the base of each toe as it is gently pulled. The practice of the movement is thus isolated, and the actions of the working hand are countered. With the working hand, pull on the toe. This is a slow, firm movement.

Go on to the next toe and repeat. Repeat with each toe.

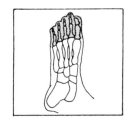

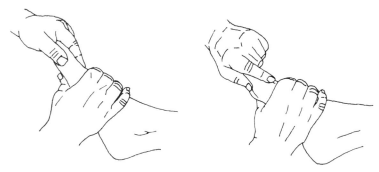

Variation:

Pull-and-turn technique
With the working hand, pull on the toe and then turn it first in a clockwise direction and then in a counterclockwise direction.

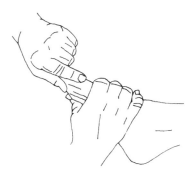

CIRCLING

The goal of the technique is to move the foot through the integrated activity of a movement in a circle. To provide variety of experience, the foot is held in one of four basic foot positions and moved in a circle.

Holding hand (L): Grasp the foot as shown and exert a slight pull on the ankle.

Working hand (R): Note the position of the working hand. In the technique as applied to Dorsiflexion and Eversion, the foot is guided primarily by the tips of the thumb and fingers. In the Inversion and Plantarflexion technique application, the palm of the hand guides the foot.

| Dorsiflexion | Eversion | Plantarflexion | Inversion |

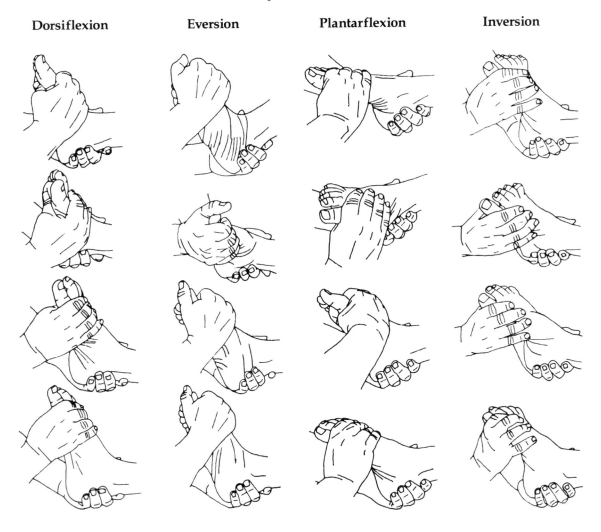

The Workout

A workout is a pattern for working through the foot in a consistent, repeatable manner. Such a pattern establishes a framework for evaluation — a system for comparing and contrasting one foot to another. Evaluation is a tool used to gather information and to determine which parts of the foot to emphasize with the application of further techniques. Evaluation determines how much time and effort should be allocated to an area.

Evaluation is based on observations made before, during, and after the application of technique. The information that is gathered is assessed on the basis of various relationships which link foot to body.

Evaluating the foot is a matter of contrast and compare. How does the foot being worked compare to other feet? Also, what have the feet been doing and how long have they been doing it? In many occupations, for example, standing for long periods is a part of the job. As a result, some foot muscles are over-used and some are under-used.

Visual and physical observations form the basis of evaluating the feet. Observations made before, during, and after the application of technique provide information to select areas for further work. Observations include both the visual and touch, locomotive, and movement. From this information a picture of the foot and its relationships emerges. Relationships within the foot and with the rest of the body provide the framework for the evaluation.

Visual and touch observations are used in the application of reflexology, stride replication®, and propriocise® techniques to determine areas for further work. Further observations are made during the application of stride application® and propriocise® techniques. These observations are, however, the basis of evaluation for reflexology and its pressure techniques.

EVALUATING THE FOOT: VISUAL AND TOUCH OBSERVATIONS

Visual Observation

A brief glance over the foot offers an opportunity to note any hangnail, ingrown nail, open cut, plantar wart, injury, or a part of the foot that may be painful or sensitive to the touch.

Further information about the foot's experiences and resulting condition is provided by looking at nails, joints, corns, callouses, bunions, and other indicators of stress.

To practice visual observation, note the characteristics of your own feet.

Comparative Elements	Characteristics
Nails	_____Thick nails
	_____Irregularly shaped nails
	_____Damaged nails
	_____Ingrown nails
Joints	_____Irregularly shaped joints
	_____Thickened joints
Foot	_____Flexibility
	_____Puffiness
	_____Injury
	_____Corn
	_____Callousing
	_____Bunion
	_____Plantar wart
	_____Arch
	_____Low
	_____High

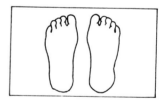

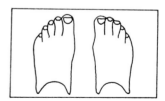

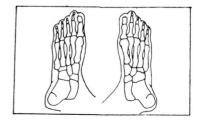

Touch as an Evaluative Tool

Working with the feet develops the sense of touch and refines one's abilities to contrast and compare. Assessment by touch is a matter of noting what one feels in various segments of the foot. To practice touch as an evaluative tool, consider your own feet.

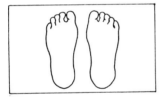

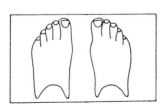

Comparative Elements	Characteristics
Fleshiness	_____Resilience, tone or texture of the felt surface
	_____Absence of muscle tone
	_____Consistency of muscle tone throughout the foot
	_____Puffiness
	_____Stringiness
Texture of the skin	_____Dryness/oiliness
	_____Perspiration
	_____Coloring
	_____Consistency of coloring throughout the foot
	_____Temperature
	_____Consistency of temperature throughout the foot
Pain tolerance	_____Sensitivity/insensitivity
	_____Consistent sensitivity throughout the foot
	_____Acute sensitivity
Under-the-surface texture	_____Buildup
	_____Puffiness

Evaluation of Visual and Touch Observations

In reflexology, visual and touch observations are evaluated on the basis of zonal, referral, and reiterative relationships which link the foot to the body.

ZONAL RELATIONSHIP

The zonal relationship notes ten equal longitudinal segments running the length of the body which conveniently match the number of toes and fingers. The basic premise is that any part of one segment affects that entire segment. By extension, the application of sensory experience to any part of the segment affects the entire segment.

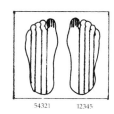
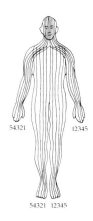

REFERRAL RELATIONSHIP

Referral relationships offer an expanded system for relating body parts; specifically the limbs. The relationship is based on the above mentioned zones. Following the basic premise, one segment of a zone affects and is affected by any other segment of the zone. Thus a segment of zone "one" in the arm relates to a segment of zone "one" in the leg.

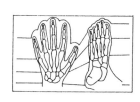
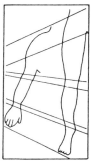

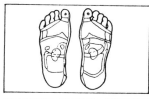

REITERATIVE RELATIONSHIP

Reiteration is a relationship in which the body whole is reflected on a body part. In reflexology, the body whole is reiterated on the hands and feet.

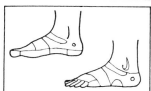

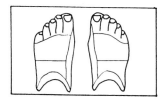

EVALUATING THE FOOT: LOCOMOTIVE OBSERVATIONS

The foot's experience is considered by judging elements of its role in locomotion. The position of the foot, the portion of the sole that meets the surface, and the foot's link to the leg through the ankle all play a role in a foot step. The foot is evaluated according to each of these characteristics during a stride replication® workout.

Quadrants of Muscular Effort

The foot's effort to position itself is the result of movement in a direction produced by the interaction of four major muscle groups. Each muscle group contributes to directional movement through its contraction and relaxation. These four major muscle groups are mirrored in quadrants of muscular effort which constitute areas for application of stride replication® techniques. (See "Positioning of the Foot".)

Each quadrant represents the muscular effort needed to re-position the foot in a particular direction. Quadrant I, for example, represents the home position of inversion or the primary muscle group needed to move the foot into an inverted position. The quadrant illustration represents the direction that the sole of the foot faces with respect to the body when the foot is placed in a home position.

Within the quadrant, the focal point provides a key area of interest. The focal point represents a part of the foot through which pass each muscle of the muscle group. Close proximity is, therefore, provided to work with the muscles of the muscle group.

Inversion is made possible by the **Muscular Effort** represented by **Quadrant I.**

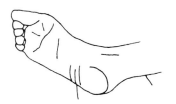 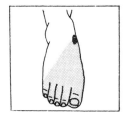 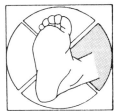

POSITIONING OF THE FOOT

Foot Position (Directional Movement)	Quadrant of Muscular Effort/Focal Point	Quadrant

I N V E R S I O N

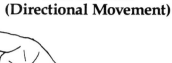
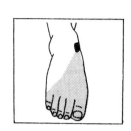
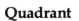
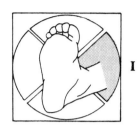

I

P L A N T A R F L E X I O N

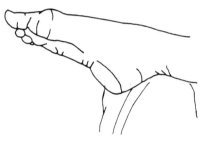
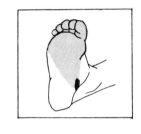
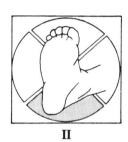

II

E V E R S I O N

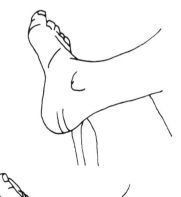
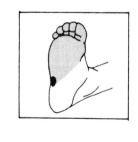
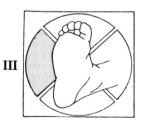

III

IV

D O R S I F L E X I O N

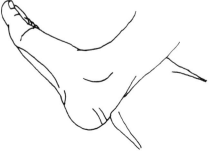
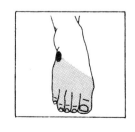
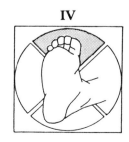

OBSERVATION BY CIRCLING TECHNIQUE

The ability of the foot to move in a direction is evaluated during the application of the circling technique. The goal of the assessment is to get a feel for the foot's ability. Does the foot feel as if it is easily being turned in a circle? Or is there a sense of resistance, a stiffness, or an inability to smoothly move in any portion of the full circle? The areas of resistance singled out form areas of interest to which certain techniques are applied. In particular, the quadrants which represent muscle groups are evaluated for their "feel" as the foot is moved through a circle.

Quadrant	Characteristics			
	Freely mobile	Impinged/ Resistant	Immobile	Response from client
I	_____	_____	_____	_____
II	_____	_____	_____	_____
III	_____	_____	_____	_____
IV	_____	_____	_____	_____

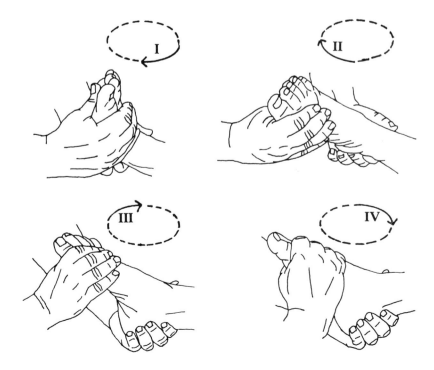

EVALUATION BY QUADRANT

In evaluation by quadrant a three stage pattern of test, apply technique, re-test is established. The foot is tested during the circling technique. It is then placed in a stretched position replicating one of four basic foot positions and the technique of cupping, tapping for percussion is applied. The foot is then re-tested to evaluate the response to the technique application.

Procedure	Assessment	Choices
Test by circling	Choose a quadrant for technique application	Quadrant I, II, III, or IV
Apply technique	Choose a technique to apply to the quadrant	Cupping, Tapping, Percussion
Re-test by circling	Feedback from re-test	Choose a quadrant and technique

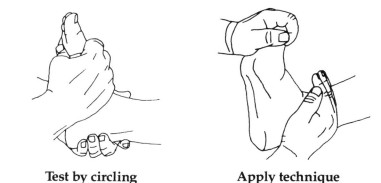

Test by circling   **Apply technique**   **Re-test by circling**

The next technique to be applied is determined by that evaluation. Is the feel of the circling foot less resistant, easier or smoother in the quadrant of the foot to which the technique has been applied? The answer to this question is considered in making further choices about which quadrant and technique to work with. The choice is to vary technique, quadrant, or both.

All quadrants cooperate to place the foot in position. This required interaction among quadrants establishes relationships upon which technique application is based. Those relationships are *continuing, neighboring,* and *opposites.*

In a continuing relationship, the application of technique to the same quadrant is made on the basis of continuing the relaxation response within one quadrant. Another technique is chosen or the same technique is applied.

The neighboring relationship recognizes the cooperation of other quadrants in the actions of a particular quadrant. Neighboring quadrants represent muscle groups which interact during a foot step.

Neighbors

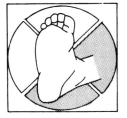 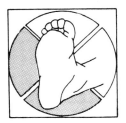 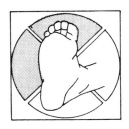 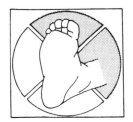

Opposing muscle groups contract and relax with respect to each other. The relationship of opposites speaks to the cooperation of these oppositional muscles in timing their actions.

Opposites

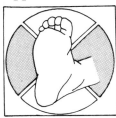 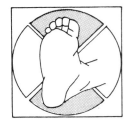

Example of Test-Apply-Re-test

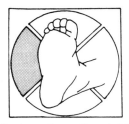 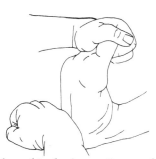

Choice of quadrant: III   **Choice of technique: Percussion**

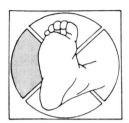

Choice of relationship: Continuing

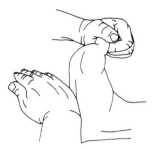

Choice of technique: Tapping

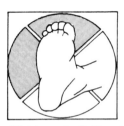

Choice of relationship: Neighboring

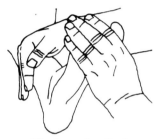

Choice of technique: Cupping

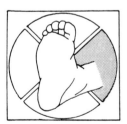

Choice of relationship: Opposites

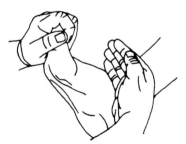

Choice of technique: Tapping

Application of Technique by Full Quadrant

Application of technique to the full quadrant and not just the focal point is a choice for course of action in evaluating through quadrant. The relationships of continuing, opposites and neighboring provide considerations for technique application.

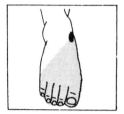 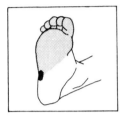 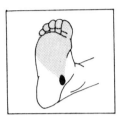 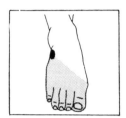

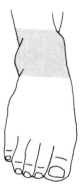

The Ankle

The ankle links leg and foot. The four major muscle groups of the foot which create directional movement pass through the ankle. The close proximity of the muscle groups in the ankle creates areas of special interest in the application of stride replication® techniques.

Sole Meets Surface

Sensors along the stride path and standing pattern receive varying amounts of pressure, and thus become areas of special interest in the application of stride replication techniques. Techniques are applied to the sole of the foot as the foot is held in a position of dorsiflexion so that the stride path is accessible for work.

To evaluate the stride path, get a feel for its resilience. As the technique is applied, the resistance of the foot to the practitioner's work is evaluated. In a similar vein, a tennis ball's bounce is judged as it is dropped on concrete. Consider the "bounce-back" of the practitioner's hand as it makes contact with the foot.

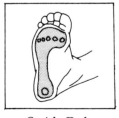

Stride Path

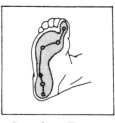

Standing Pattern

Foot: _____Springs back

_____Give and take

_____Deadens the bounce

EVALUATING THE FOOT: MOVEMENT OBSERVATIONS

A propriocise® workout is an on-going evaluation of the foot's response to technique application. Responses are an indication of the foot's experience including accident, injury, extreme stress, accumulated stress, prolonged illness, and/or the role of the foot at work or play.

The joints themselves are not responsible for their own movement. They participate in shaping intended movement and, as such, become the focus of propriocise® techniques. The joints transform the stress of muscular tension into motion, translating force into action. Adaptations necessary for locomotion occur at the joints. The stress of experience placed upon the joint determine its structure and its ability to perform.

Compensation for the stress of both limited and overly practiced movements is the focus of propriocise® techniques. The techniques target individual joints and their range of movement as well as integrated movements of the whole foot. Integrated movements are those in which several foot positions are combined to replicate the foot's positioning in a foot step.

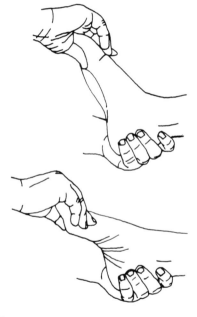

The opposite movements of dorsiflexion and plantar-flexion, for example, are the focus of one technique. This consideration of opposite foot position provides evaluation material for the practitioner and experience of range of motion for the foot. Movement in neighboring foot positions provides additional information. The characteristics displayed by the foot during technique application inform one of the flexibility of the foot.

Movement of the foot is compared and contrasted during a propriocise® workout. The part of the foot being worked is evaluated for its ability to move when compared with:

- the foot's full potential
- one joint to another
- one part of the foot to another
- the same segment in both feet
- the foot to other feet you've worked on
- the foot to your own.

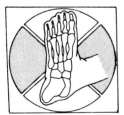
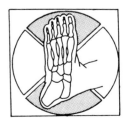

Opposites

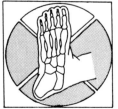

Neighboring

Quadrant	Characteristics			
	Freely mobile	Impinged/ Resistant	Immobile	Response from client
Opposites I/III	_____	_____	_____	_____
II/IV Neighboring I/II/III	_____	_____	_____	_____
III/IV/I	_____	_____	_____	_____

Movement Observations

The feel of the movement performed by the technique in propriocise® indicates the ability of the joint to move. Characteristics of flexibility are observed, during the application of the technique. To practice movement observations, note the characteristics of your own feet.

Comparative Element   **Characteristic**

Flexibility   _____Stiffness

_____Swelling

_____Consistent flexibility

_____Snap, crackle, and pop

_____Unstressed (neutral client response)

_____Stressed (negative client response)

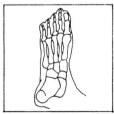
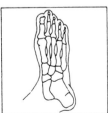

The Workouts

FIVE-MINUTE FOOT LOOSENER (Workout)

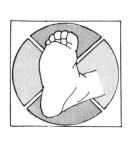

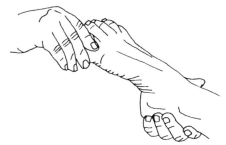

Foot flicking/toes,
page 48

Side to side,
page 45

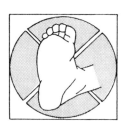

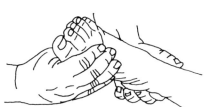

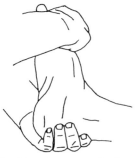

Circling (clockwise)
page 27

Circling (counterclockwise)
page 28

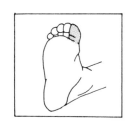

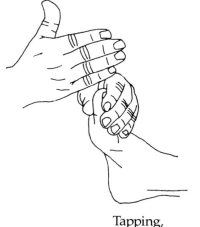

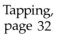

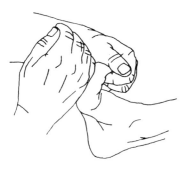

Tapping,
page 32

Tapping,
page 32

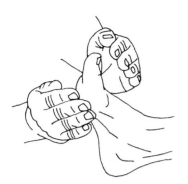

Cupping, page 35

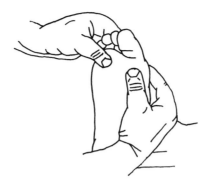

Metatarsal grasp, page 50

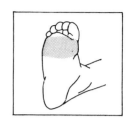

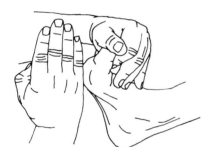

Tapping, page 32

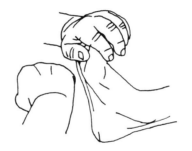

Percussion, page 30

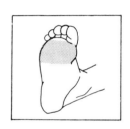

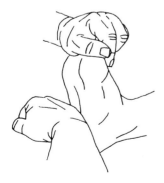

Percussion, page 30

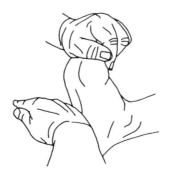

Tapping, page 32

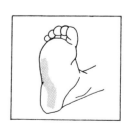

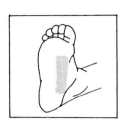
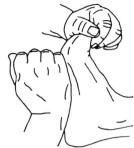
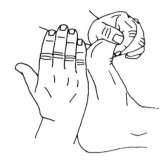

Percussion, page 30

Tapping, page 32

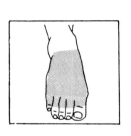
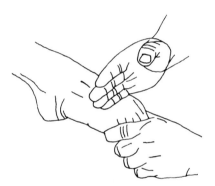
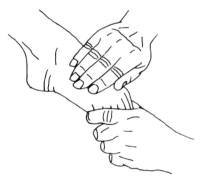

Tapping, page 32

Cupping, page 35

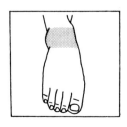
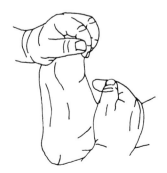
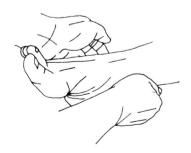

Cupping, page 35

Cupping, page 35

THE COMPLETE WORKOUT

Side to side, page 45

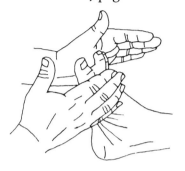 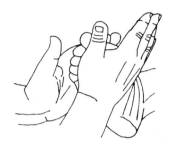 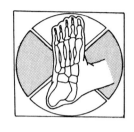

Tapping, page 32

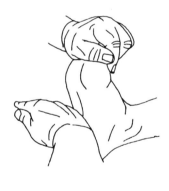 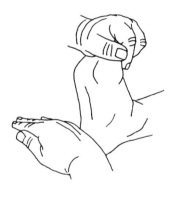 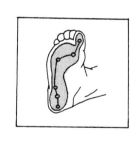

Foot flicking, page 48

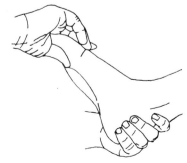 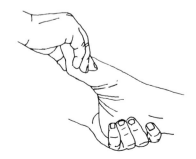 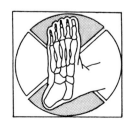

Circling (plantarflexion), page 27

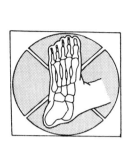

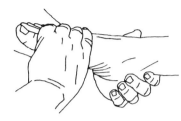

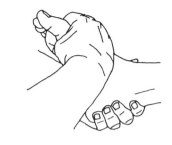

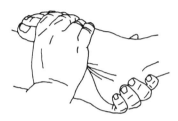

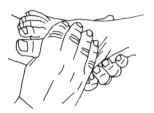

Tapping, page 32

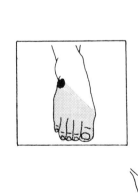

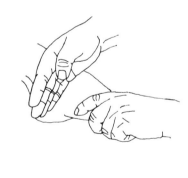

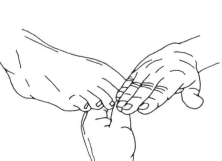

Metatarsal fan, page 44

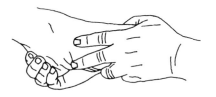 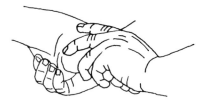 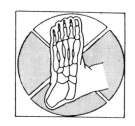

Tapping, page 32

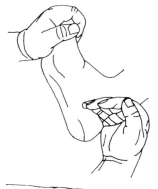 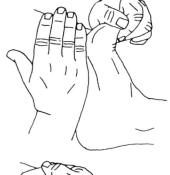

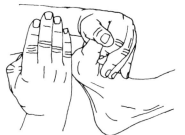 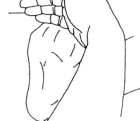 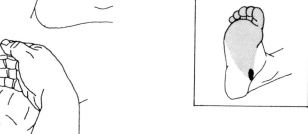

Percussion, page 30

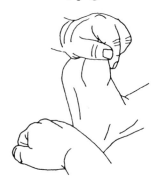 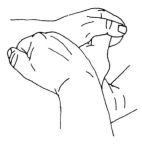 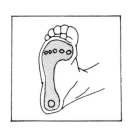

Metatarsal grasp, page 50

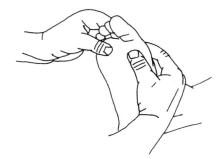

Metatarsal fan, page 44

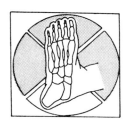
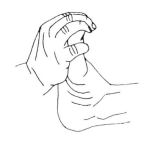
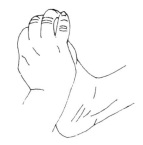

Circling (inversion), page 27

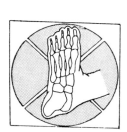
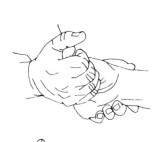
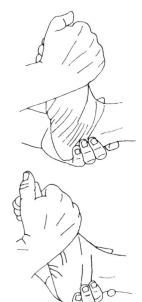
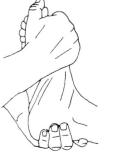

Tapping, page 32

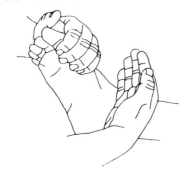 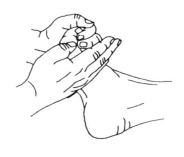 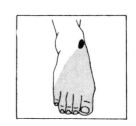

Cupping, page 35   **Tapping,** page 32

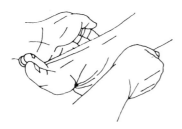 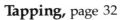 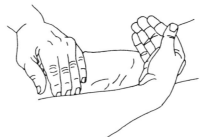 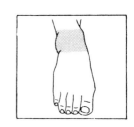

Side to side, page 45

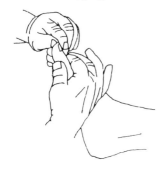 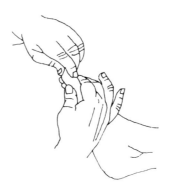 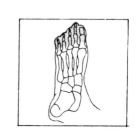

Heel to toe mover, page 46

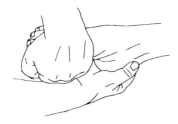 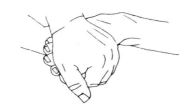 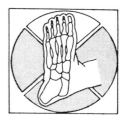

Circling (dorsiflexion), page 27

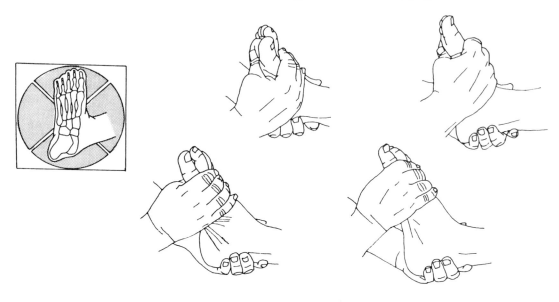

Percussion, page 30

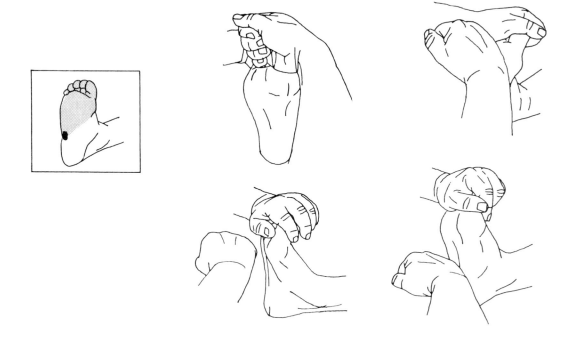

Plantar rocker, page 47

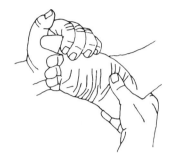 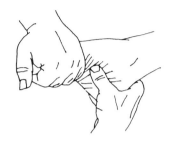 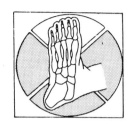

Metatarsal lever, page 49

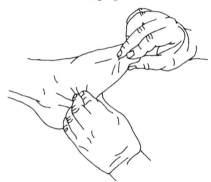 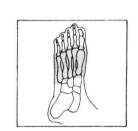

Cupping, page 35

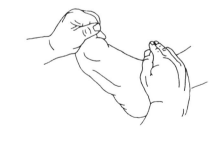 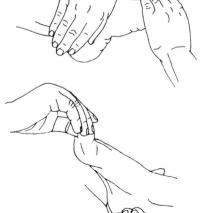 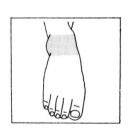

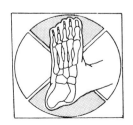

STRIDE REPLICATION® WORKOUT

In the Stride Replication® Workout, each routine or technique series begins and ends with a test by circling. Following a test the possibilities for further technique application are the technique series; full quadrant, opposites, neighboring, and ankle. (See "The Workout," page 53, "Special Interests," page 105 .)

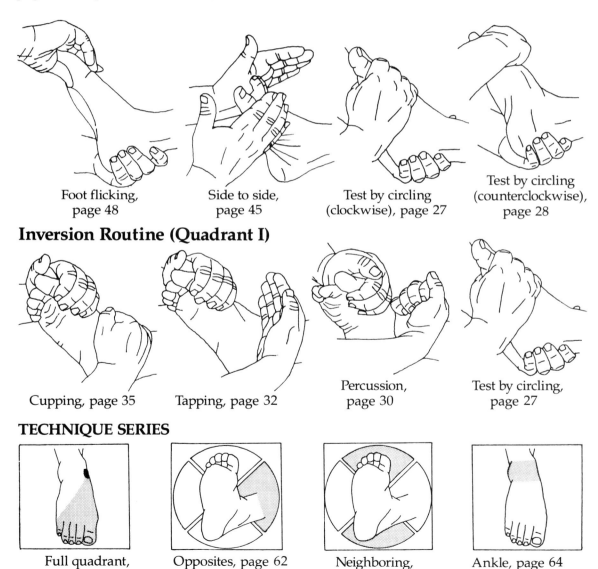

Foot flicking, page 48

Side to side, page 45

Test by circling (clockwise), page 27

Test by circling (counterclockwise), page 28

Inversion Routine (Quadrant I)

Cupping, page 35

Tapping, page 32

Percussion, page 30

Test by circling, page 27

TECHNIQUE SERIES

Full quadrant, page 61

Opposites, page 62

Neighboring, page 62

Ankle, page 64

Plantarflexion Routine (Quadrant II)

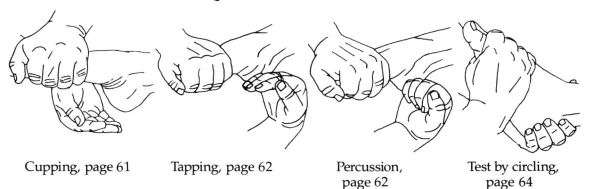

Cupping, page 61   Tapping, page 62   Percussion, page 62   Test by circling, page 64

TECHNIQUE SERIES

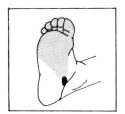 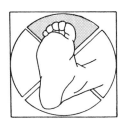 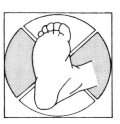 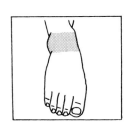

Full quadrant, page 35   Opposites, page 32   Neighboring, page 30   Ankle, page 27

Eversion Routine (Quadrant III)

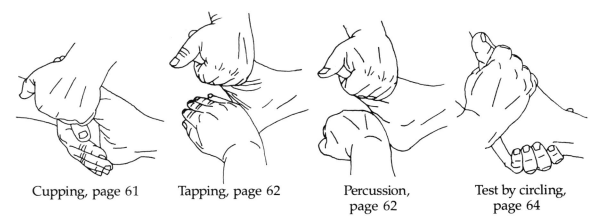

Cupping, page 61   Tapping, page 62   Percussion, page 62   Test by circling, page 64

TECHNIQUE SERIES

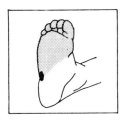

Full quadrant,
page 61

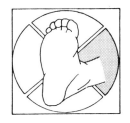

Opposites, page 62

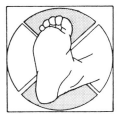

Neighboring,
page 62

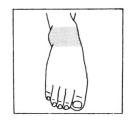

Ankle, page 64

Dorsiflexion Routine (Quadrant IV)

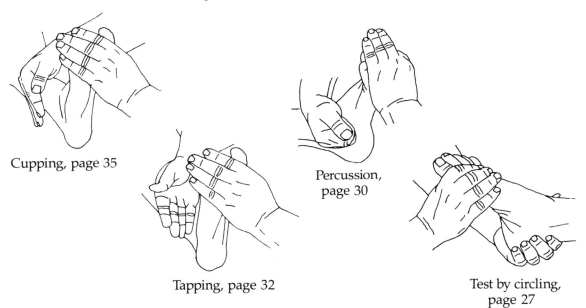

Cupping, page 35

Tapping, page 32

Percussion,
page 30

Test by circling,
page 27

TECHNIQUE SERIES

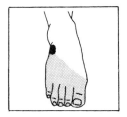

Full quadrant,
page 61

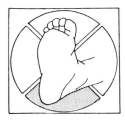

Opposites, page 62

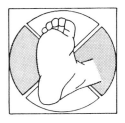

Neighboring,
page 62

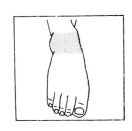

Ankle, page 64

PROPRIOCISE® WORKOUT

H: Indicates instructions for the holding hand.
W(R): Indicates instructions for the working right hand.
W(L): Indicates instructions for the working left hand.

Side to side, page 45

H/W: Both hands play an equal role. The left hand moves the foot toward the subject while the right hand draws the foot toward the practitioner. A turning of the foot from side to side establishes a rhythmic movement of the foot.

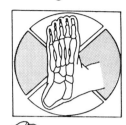

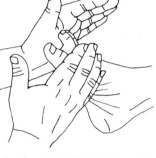

Foot flicking, page 48

H: Cup the heel of the foot. Pull slightly at the ankle.

W(R): Push with the flat of the thumb and then the flats of the fingers to create a rapid up and down movement of the foot.

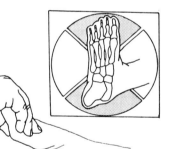

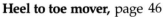

Heel to toe mover, page 46

H: Cup the heel of the foot.

W(L): Push with the heel of the working hand and holding hand. Establish a rhythmic side to side movement of the foot.

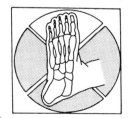

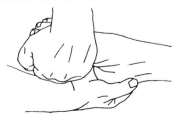

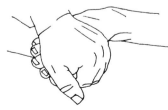

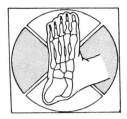

Side to side mover, page 50
H: Grasp the foot to steady it.
W(R): Grasp the foot. Push with the flat of the thumb and then the flats of the fingers to create a side to side movement of the foot.

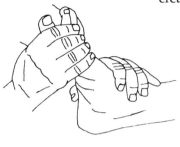
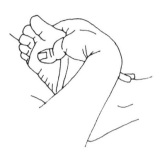

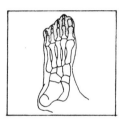

Side to side, page 45
H: Grip the joint of the toe.
W(L): Grip the tip of the toe. Move the toe from side to side.

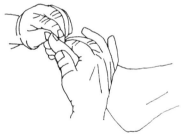
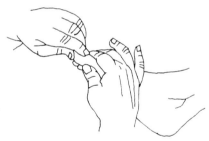

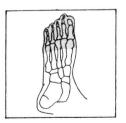

Pull and turn, page 51
H: Grasp the foot.
W(L): Grasp the toe, pull slowly, and turn gently.

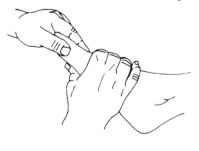
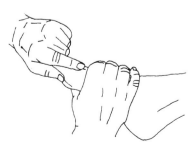

Metatarsal fan, page 44
H: At rest
W(R): Fan the heel of the hand across the metatarsal heads of the foot and back again in a countermovement.

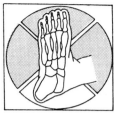

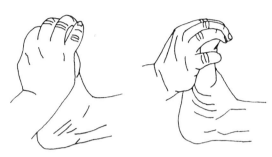

Metatarsal fan, page 44
H: Cup the heel of the foot.
W(R): Fan the heel of the hand across the metatarsal heads of the foot and back again in a countermovement.

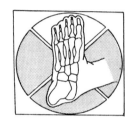

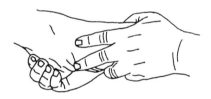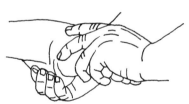

Plantar rocker, page 47
H: Cup the heel of the foot. Place the flat of the thumb at the base of the metatarsal.
W(L): Bring the foot to a toes pointed position. Roll the palm of the hand from heel to base of fingers across the metatarsls. Create a pattern of movement/countermovement.

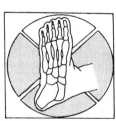

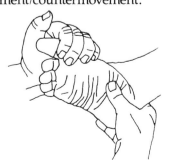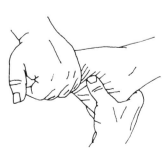

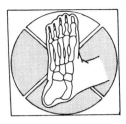

Heel to toe mover, page 46

H: Cup the foot in the heel of the hand.

W(L): Push with the heel of the hand and pull with the fingers of the holding hand. Create a pattern of movement/countermovement.

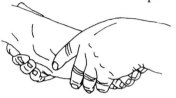
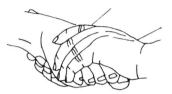

Metatarsal lever, page 49

H: Position the thumb and fingers at the base of the metatarsal. Counter the actions of the working hand.

W(R): Position the thumb and fingers at the metatarsal head. Push with the flat of the thumb and the flat of the holding fingers. Create a pattern of movement/counter-movement.

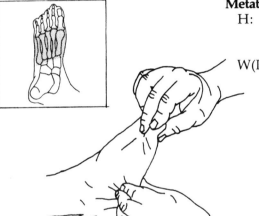

Metatarsal grasp, page 50

H/W: Both hands play an equal role. Grasp the metatarsal head. Push with the flat of the thumb (right hand) and the flats of the fingers (left hand). Create a pattern of movement/countermovement.

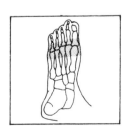

The Workout Workbook

In evaluating the foot during the workout, visual observations are made, touch and movement evaluations are noted, and the experiences of the foot are considered. "The Workout Workbook" includes a summary of evaluation information and illustrations on which to note the observations and evaluations.

EVALUATING THE FOOT

1. Visual/Touch Observations

VISUAL OBSERVATION

Nails

_____Thick nails

_____Irregularly shaped nails

_____Damaged nails

_____Ingrown nails

Joints

_____Thickened joints

_____Irregularly shaped joints

_____Flexibility of joint

Puffiness _____

Injury _____

Corn _____

Callousing _____

Bunion _____

Plantar wart _____

Arch _____

       high _____

       low _____

TOUCH AS AN EVALUATIVE TOOL

Fleshiness

_____Resilience, tone, or texture of the felt surface

_____Absence of muscle tone

_____Consistency of muscle tone throughout the foot

_____Puffiness

_____Stringiness

Texture of the skin

_____Dryness/oiliness

_____Perspiration

_____Coloring

_____Consistency of coloring throughout the foot

_____Temperature

_____Consistency of temperature throughout the foot

Pain tolerance

_____Sensitivity/insensitivity

_____Consistent sensitivity throughout the foot

_____Acute sensitivity

Under-the-surface texture

_____Buildup

_____Puffiness

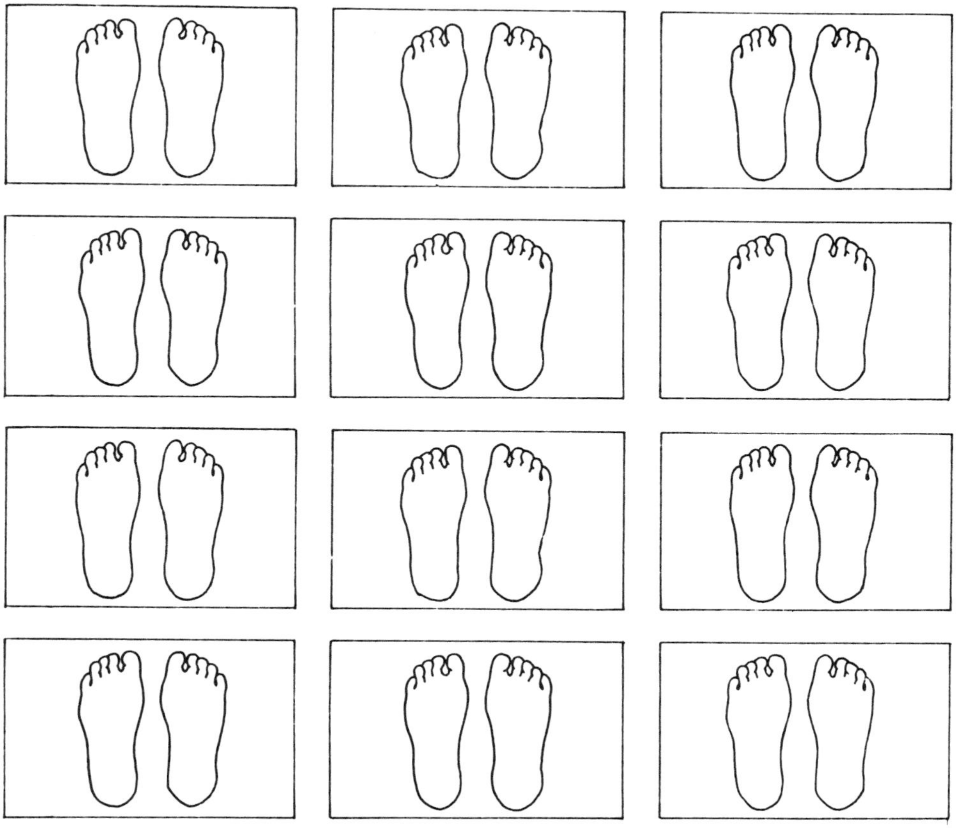

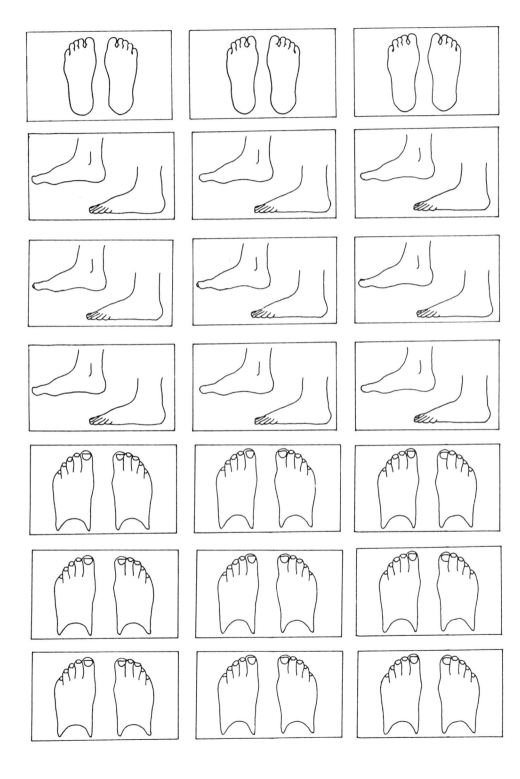

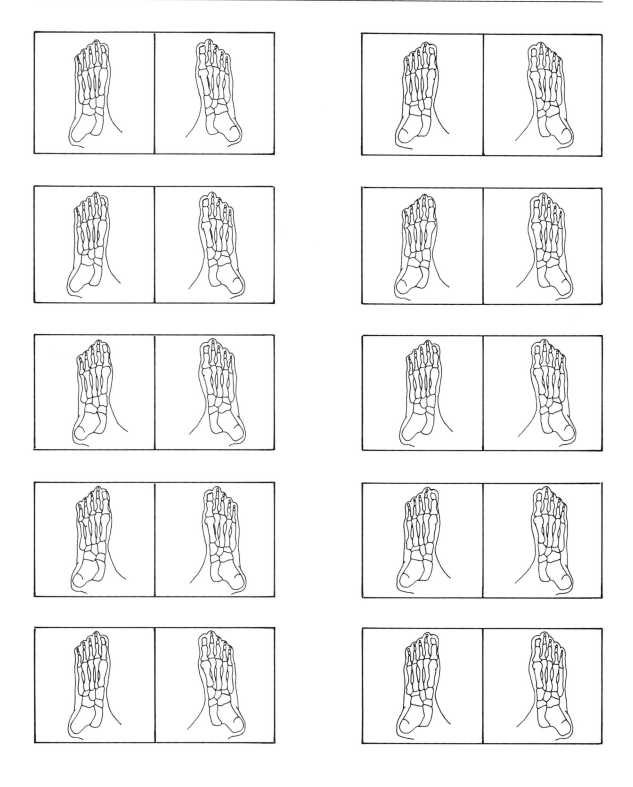

Relating Observation to Relationship

1. In which zone does the visual/touch observation occur?
2. Is there a notable referral relationship?
3. In which reiterative area does the visual/touch observation occur?

ZONAL RELATIONSHIP

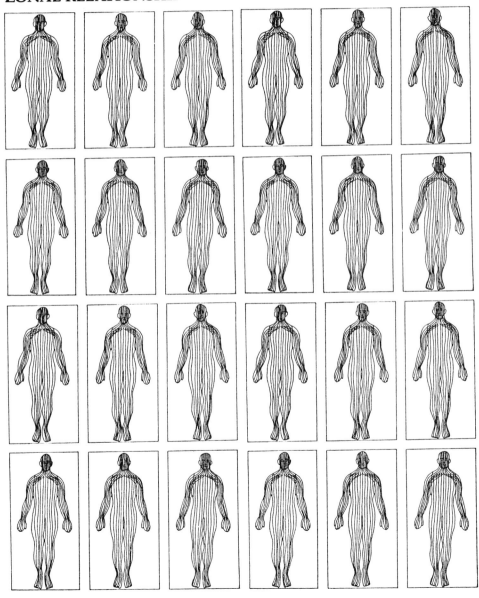

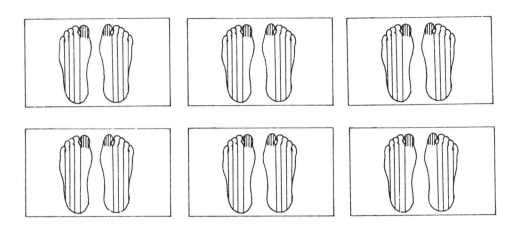

REFERRAL RELATIONSHIP

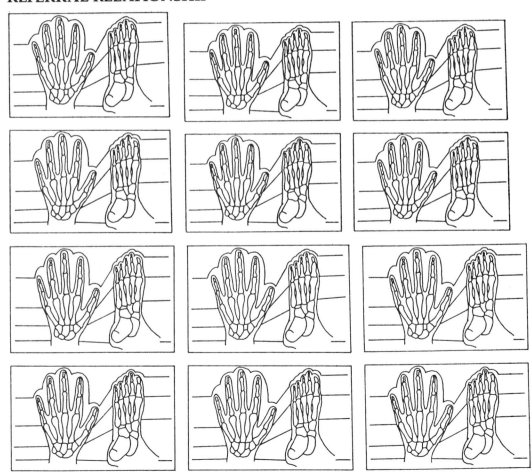

REITERATIVE RELATIONSHIP

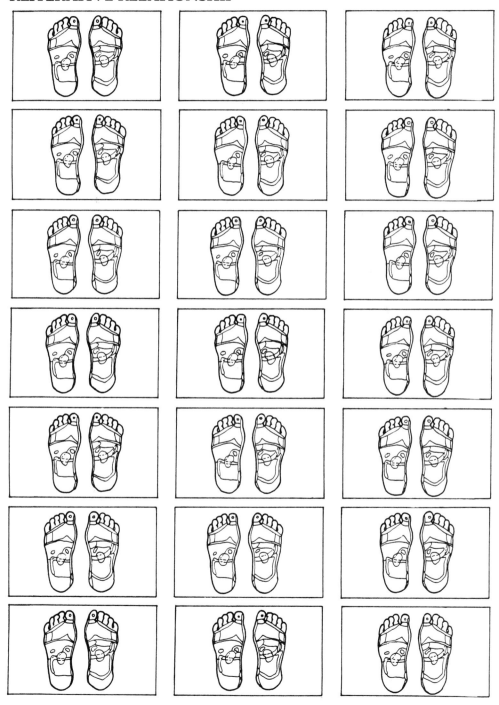

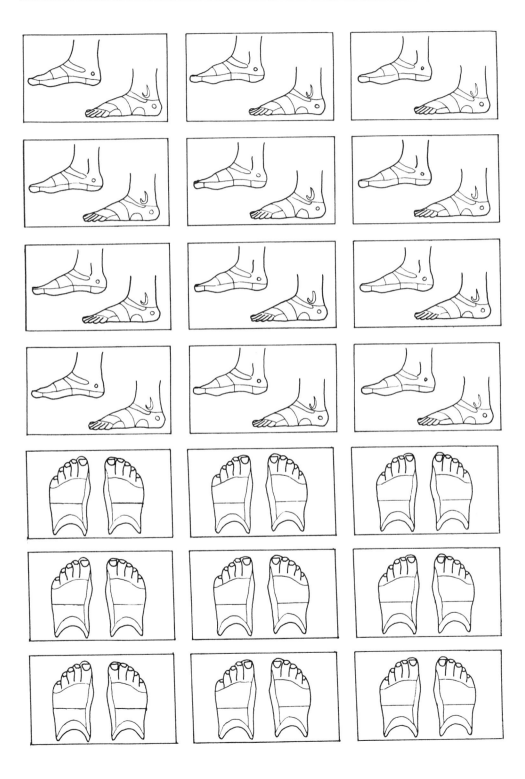

2. LOCOMOTIVE OBSERVATIONS

CIRCLING TECHNIQUE OBSERVATIONS

Characteristics	Quadrant			
	I	II	III	IV
Freely mobile	____	____	____	____
Impinged/Resistant	____	____	____	____
Immobile	____	____	____	____
Response from client	____	____	____	____

STRIDE PATH/STANDING PATTERN OBSERVATIONS

_____Springs back

_____Give and take

_____Deadens the bounce

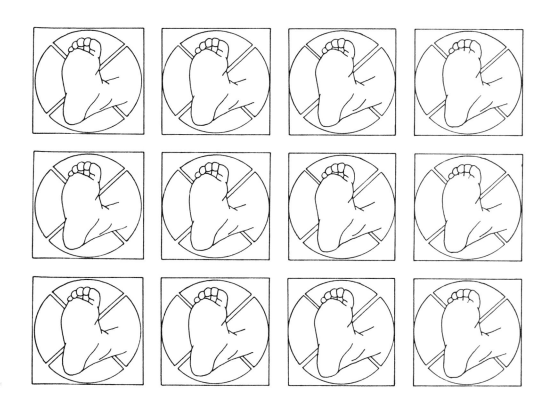

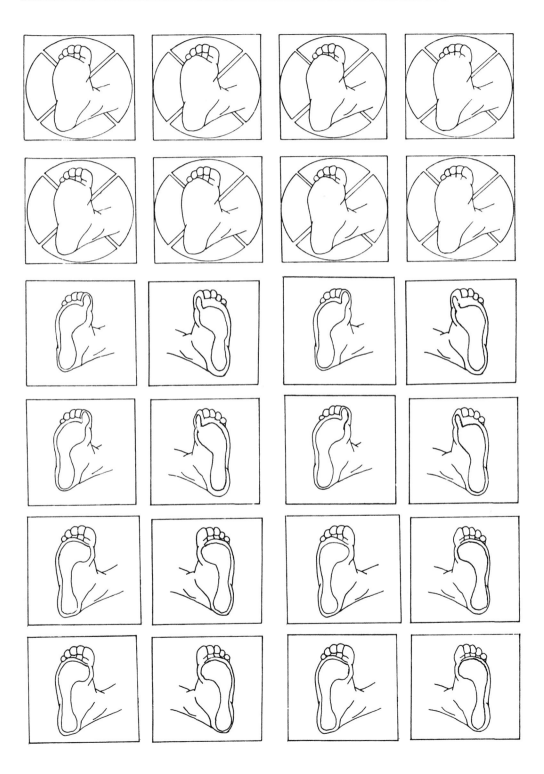

Relating Observation to Relationship

1. Which focal point and/or full quadrant is the choice for application of further techniques?

2. Is the relationship of opposites a choice for the application of further techniques?

3. Is the neighboring relationship a choice for the application of further techniques?

QUADRANT/FOCAL POINT

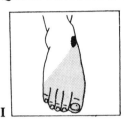 I

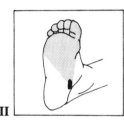 II

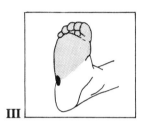 III

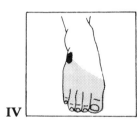 IV

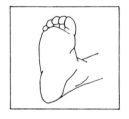

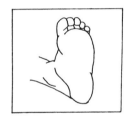

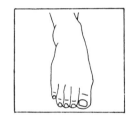

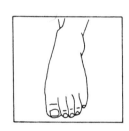

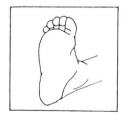

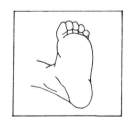

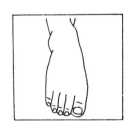

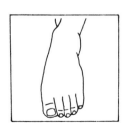

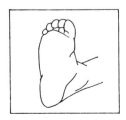

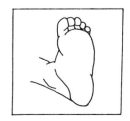

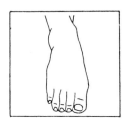

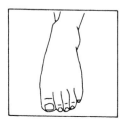

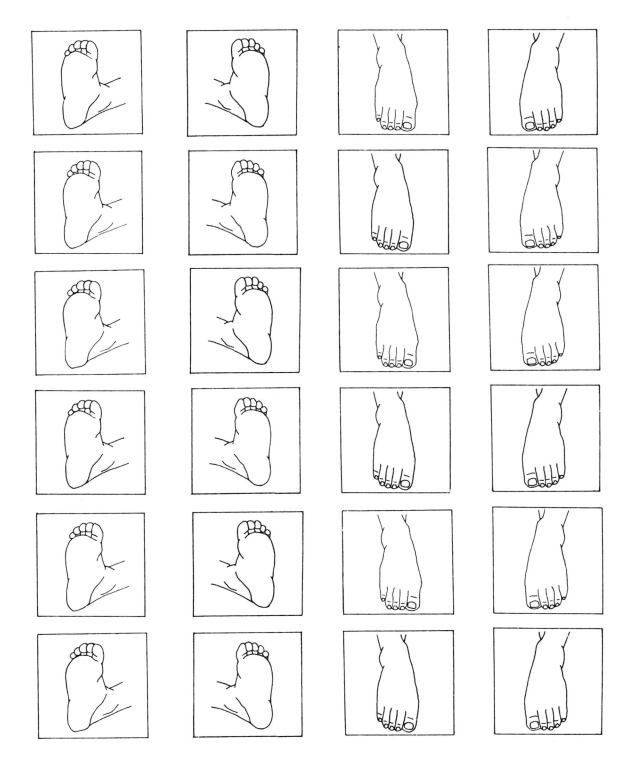

RELATIONSHIP OF OPPOSITES

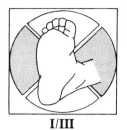

I/III

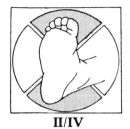

II/IV

Neighboring Relationship

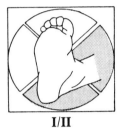

I/II

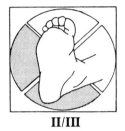

II/III

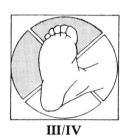

III/IV

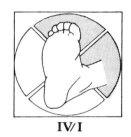

IV/I

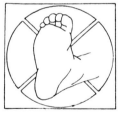
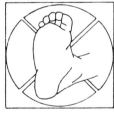
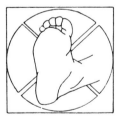
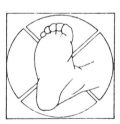

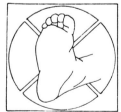
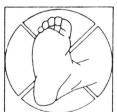
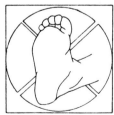
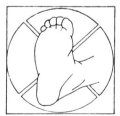

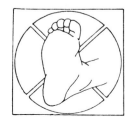
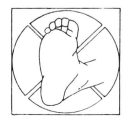
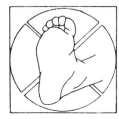
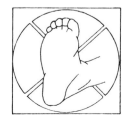

3. MOVEMENT OBSERVATIONS

Flexibility

_____Stiffness

_____Swelling

_____Consistent flexibility

_____Snap, crackle, and pop

     _____Unstressed

     _____Distressed

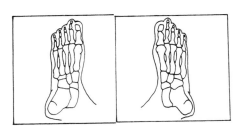
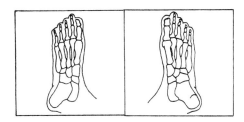

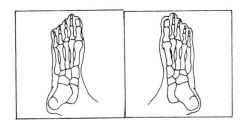
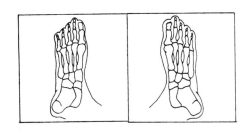

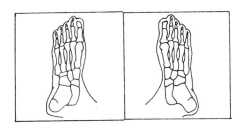
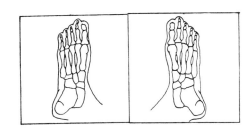

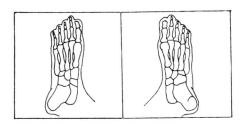
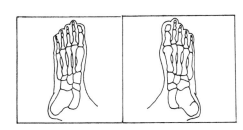

Integrated Movement Observations

Characteristics	Quadrant			
	I	II	III	IV
Freely mobile	___	___	___	___
Impinged/Resistant	___	___	___	___
Immobile	___	___	___	___
Response from client	___	___	___	___

RELATING OPPOSITES

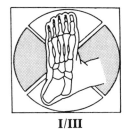
I/III

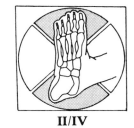
II/IV

RELATING NEIGHBORS

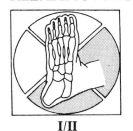
I/II

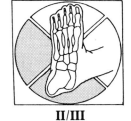
II/III

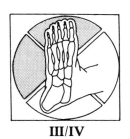
III/IV

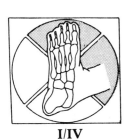
I/IV

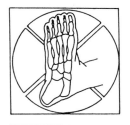

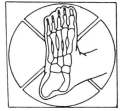

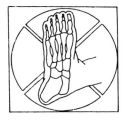

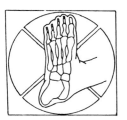

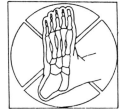

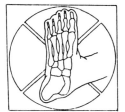

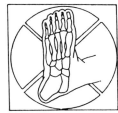

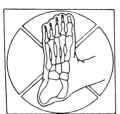

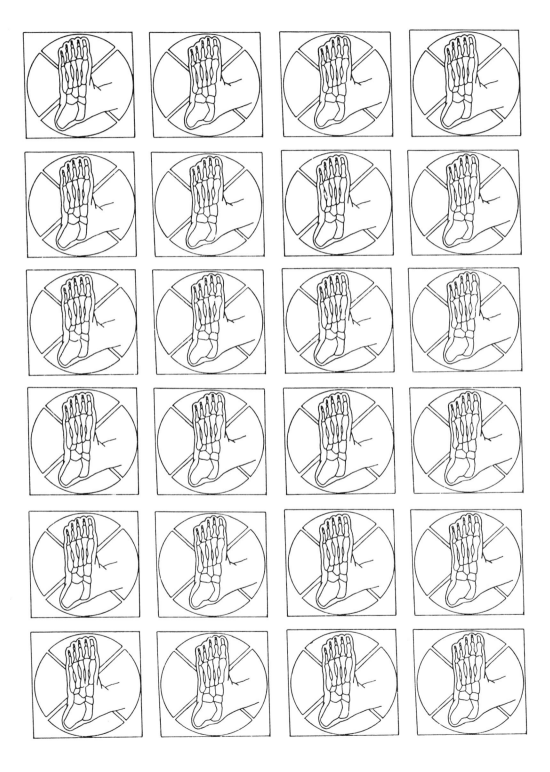

Evaluating the Feet: Summary

1. VISUAL/TOUCH OBSERVATIONS

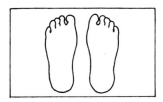 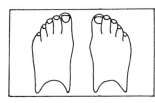 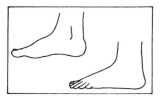

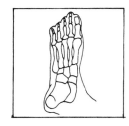 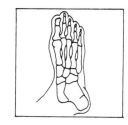

Relating Observation to Relationship

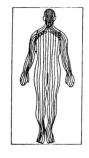 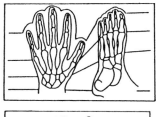 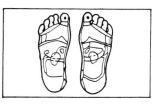 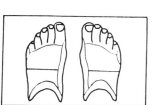

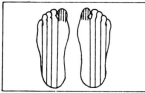 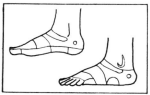

2. LOCOMOTIVE OBSERVATIONS

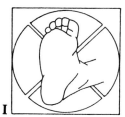 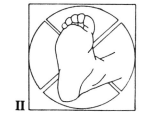 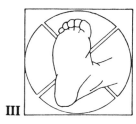 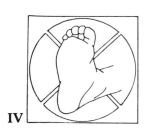

I II III IV

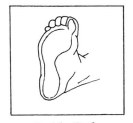
Stride Path

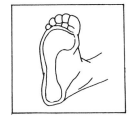
Standing Path

Relating Observation to Relationship
FOCAL POINT/QUADRANT

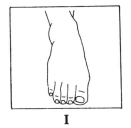
I

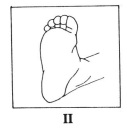
II

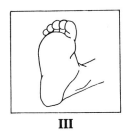
III

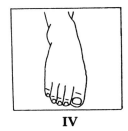
IV

OPPOSITES

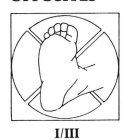
I/III

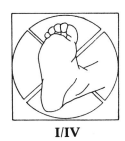
I/IV

NEIGHBORING

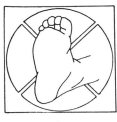
I/II

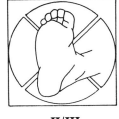
II/III

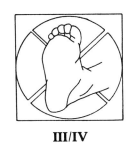
III/IV

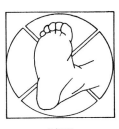
I/IV

3. MOVEMENT OBSERVATIONS
Flexibility

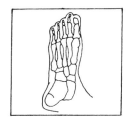 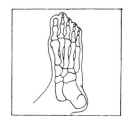

Integrated Movement
RELATING OPPOSITES

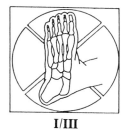
I/III

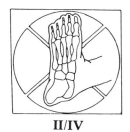
II/IV

RELATING NEIGHBORS

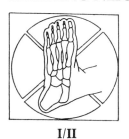
I/II

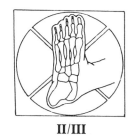
II/III

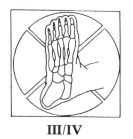
III/IV

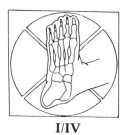
I/IV

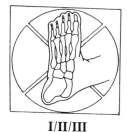
I/II/III

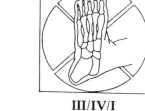
III/IV/I

Special Interests

Special Interests: Stride Replication®

"Special Interests: Stride Replication® " recognizes the role of the foot in locomotion. Areas of special interest and relationships are created by the role of the foot in meeting the surface, making directional changes, and linking with the leg through the ankle. Stride replication® techniques are applied to these areas on the basis of locomotive relationships for the purpose of interrupting the stress of walking and standing.

Each chart series in "Special Interests: Stride Replication® " notes information relevant to an area of specific interest as well as a summary of techniques applied to the area. A summary of relationship outlines the principles of technique application. The focus of technique application is noted in each chart series; "Stride Path," "Focal Point by Position," "Quadrants," and "Ankle."

Symbols and illustrations are utilized in each chart series to indicate an area of special interest and/or relationship. The information conveyed by these symbols is explained in the following material.

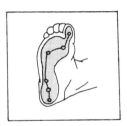

Stride Path: The portion of the foot which meets the surface in walking. Sensors which key movement are noted.

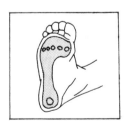

Standing Pattern: The portion of the foot which meets the surface in standing. Sensors through which weight is distributed during standing are noted.

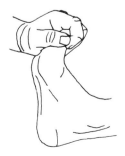

Position: The placement of the foot which mimics one of the four basic directional movements.

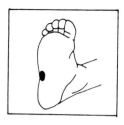

Focal point: A reflection of the muscle insertion of the muscle group needed to move the foot in a direction.

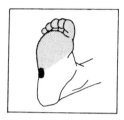

Quadrant: A representation of the muscular effort needed to move the foot in a direction.

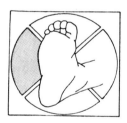

The direction that the sole of the foot faces with respect to the body when placed in position.

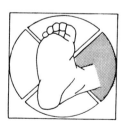

Relationship of Opposites: Opposing muscle groups contract and relax with respect to each other. The relationship of opposites speaks to the cooperation of these oppositional muscles in timing actions.

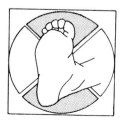

Neighboring Relationship: Recognizes the cooperation of other quadrants in the actions of a particular quadrant. Neighboring quadrants represent muscle groups which interface during a foot step.

STRIDE PATH

The foot is placed in position and a technique is then applied to the stride path. Sensors along the stride path are the focus of technique application as well as the sensors of the standing pattern.

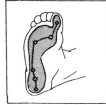 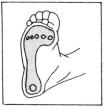

Stride Path   Standing Pattern

Technique: Percussion, page 30

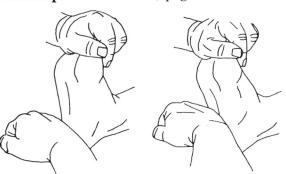 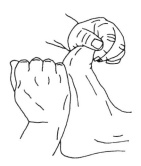 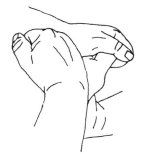

Technique: Tapping, page 32

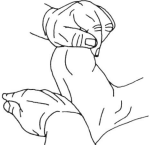 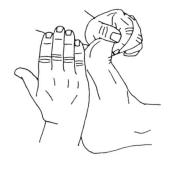

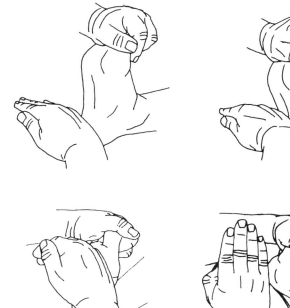 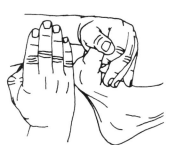 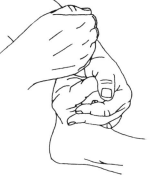

Technique: Feathering, See Kunz and Kunz, *The Complete Guide to Foot Reflexology,* Prentice-Hall, Inc., 1982.

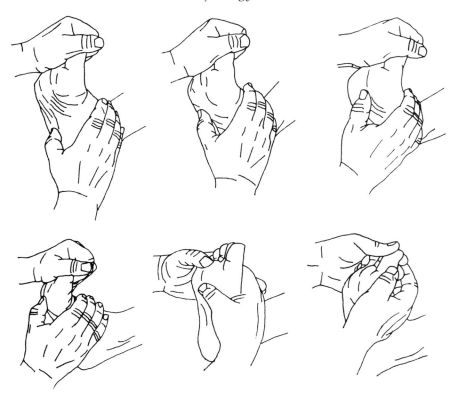

FOCAL POINT BY POSITION

A foot is placed in position and a technique is then applied to the focal point of a quadrant. "Focal Point by Position" notes the variety of sensation which may be applied to a focal point of interest. (See the techniques in the same horizontal row.) Neighboring relationships are noted. (See the techniques in the adjacent row. I and IV are "adjacent" to each other as well.) To see relationships of opposites look at every other row.

Position: Inversion

Relationships:

IV
Neighbor

Opposite
III

**Home
Position**
I

Neighbor
II

TECHNIQUE

Cupping	Tapping	Percussion	

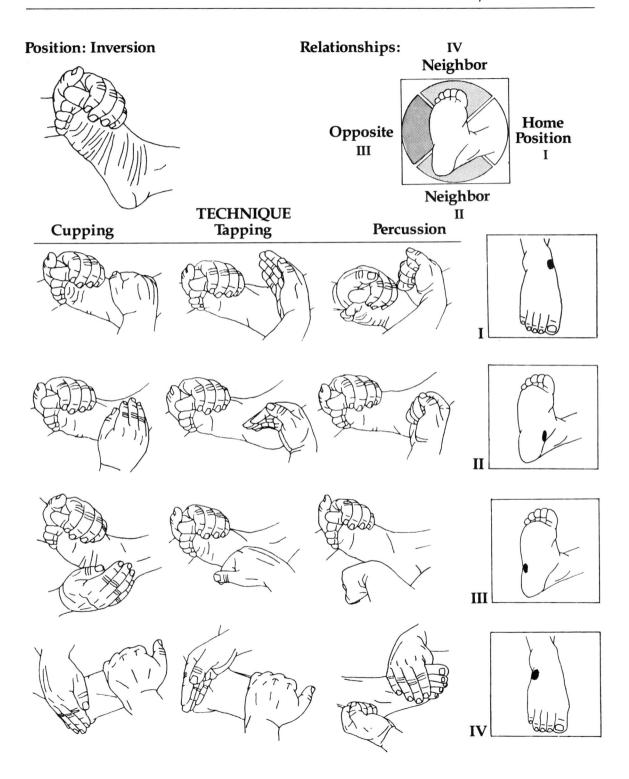

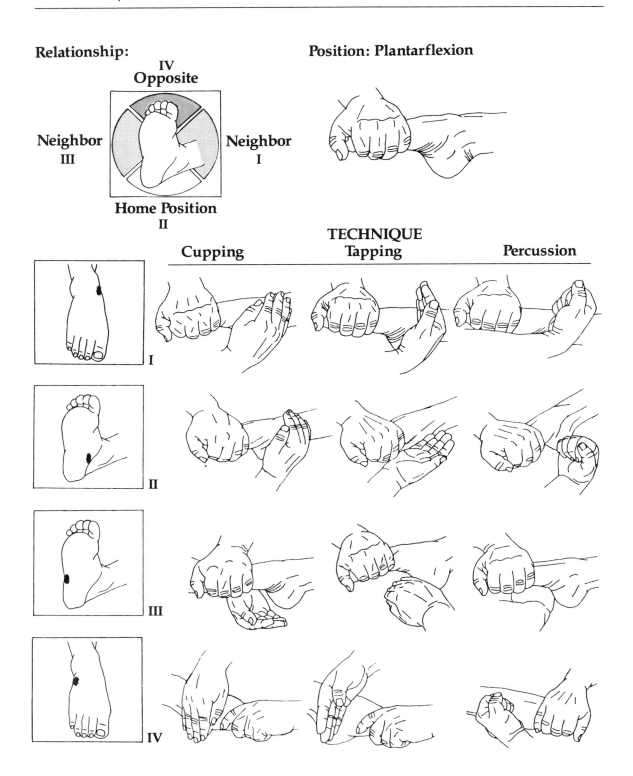

Relationship:

IV
Opposite

Neighbor
III

Neighbor
I

Home Position
II

Position: Plantarflexion

TECHNIQUE

Cupping Tapping Percussion

I

II

III

IV

Position: Eversion

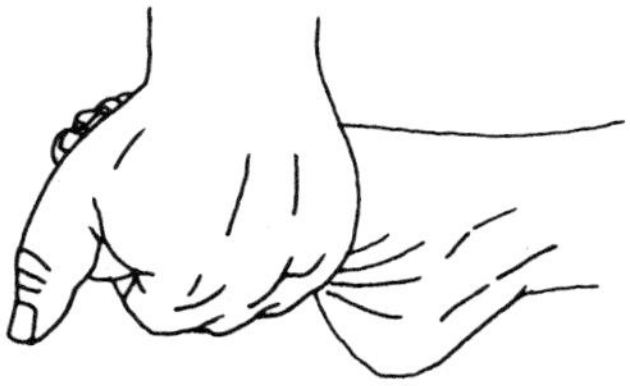

Relationships:

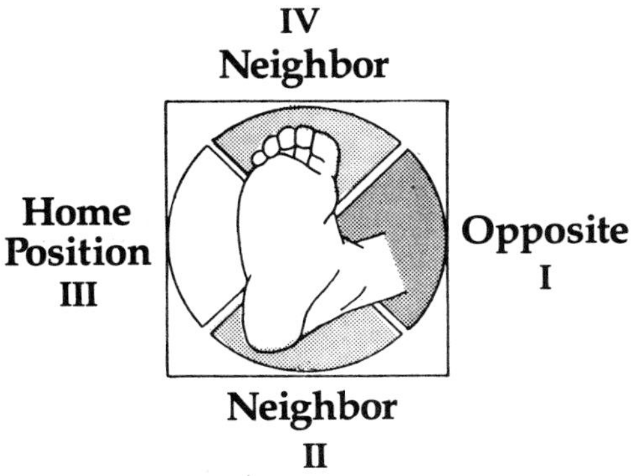

IV
Neighbor

**Home
Position
III**

**Opposite
I**

**Neighbor
II**

TECHNIQUES

Cupping	Tapping	Percussion

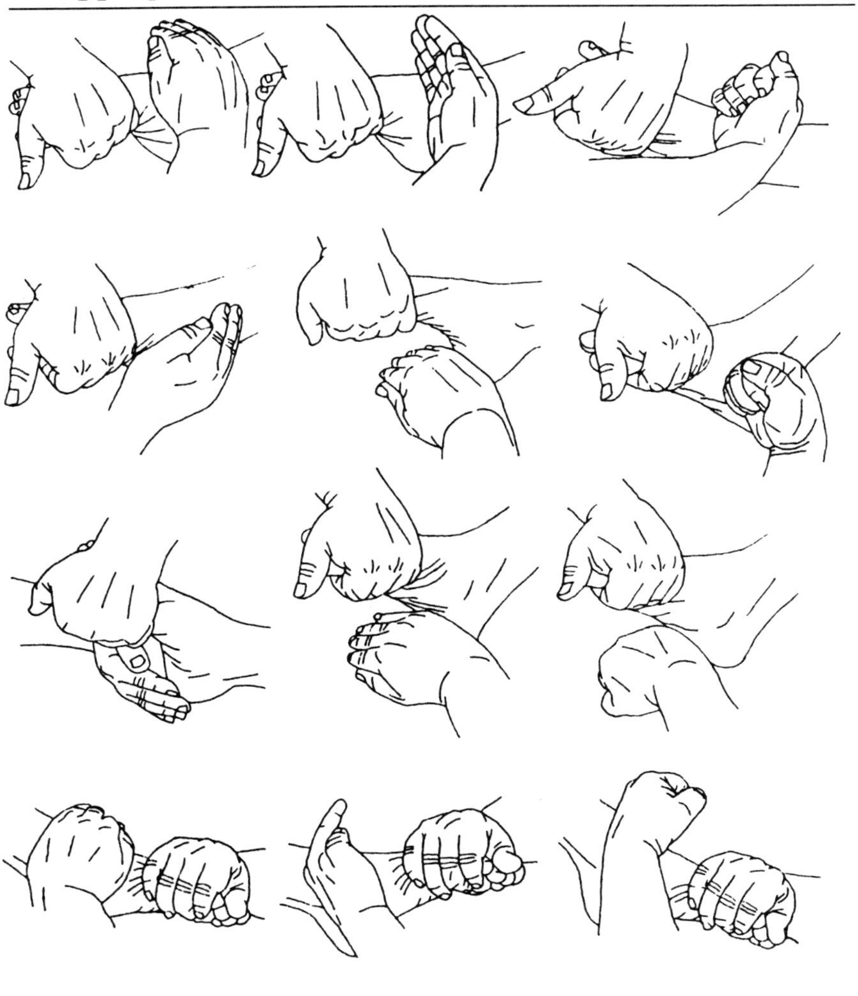

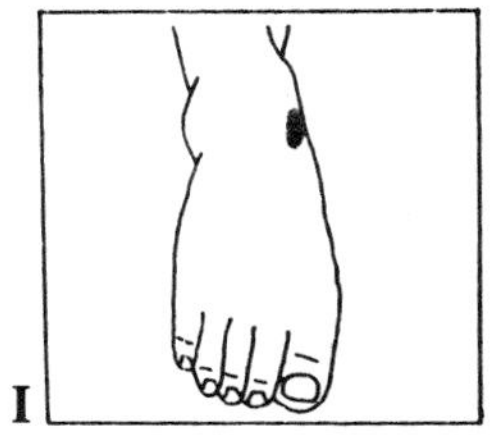

I

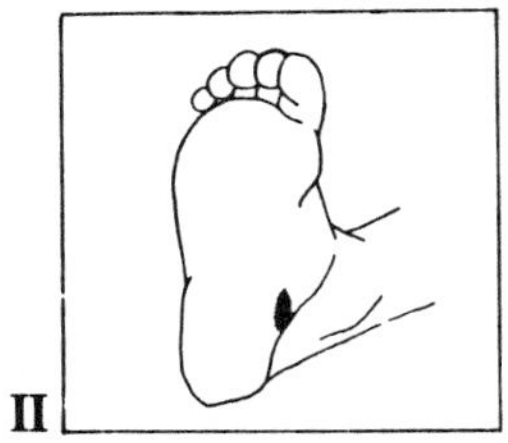

II

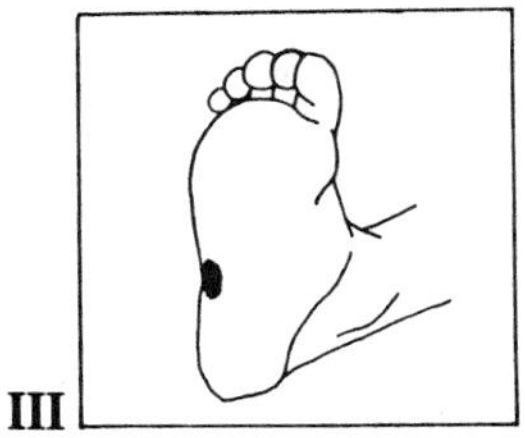

III

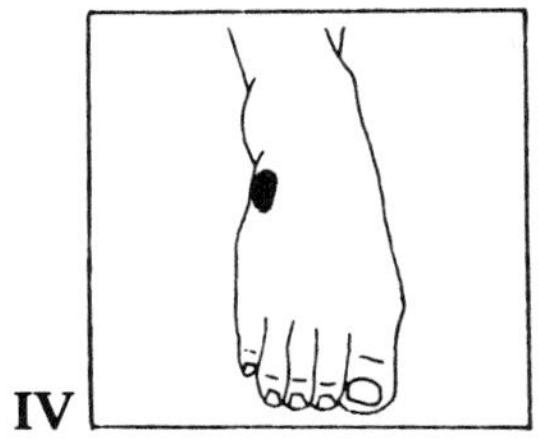

IV

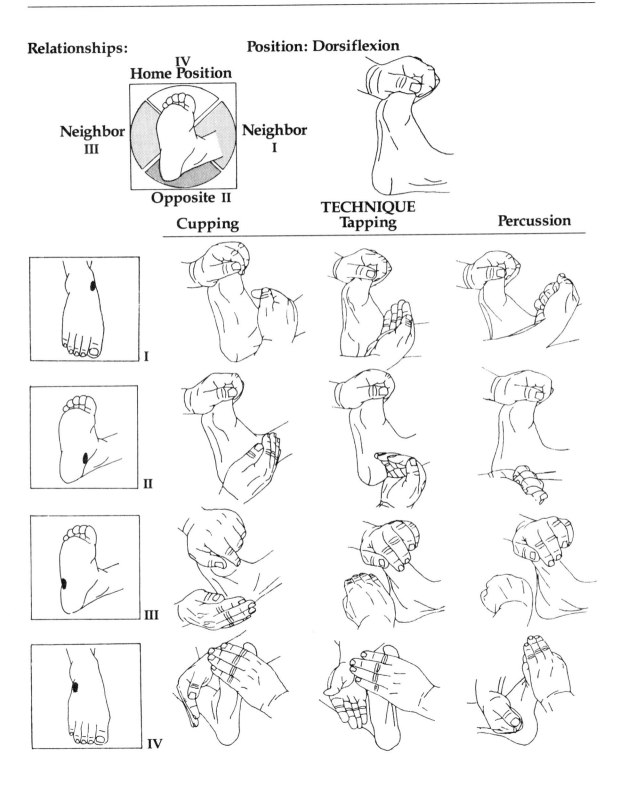

Relationships:

IV
Home Position

Neighbor
III

Neighbor
I

Opposite II

Position: Dorsiflexion

TECHNIQUE

Cupping   Tapping   Percussion

I

II

III

IV

QUADRANTS

The foot is placed in a position where the quadrant is accessible and a technique is then applied to a focal point and then the entire quadrant.

Quadrant I

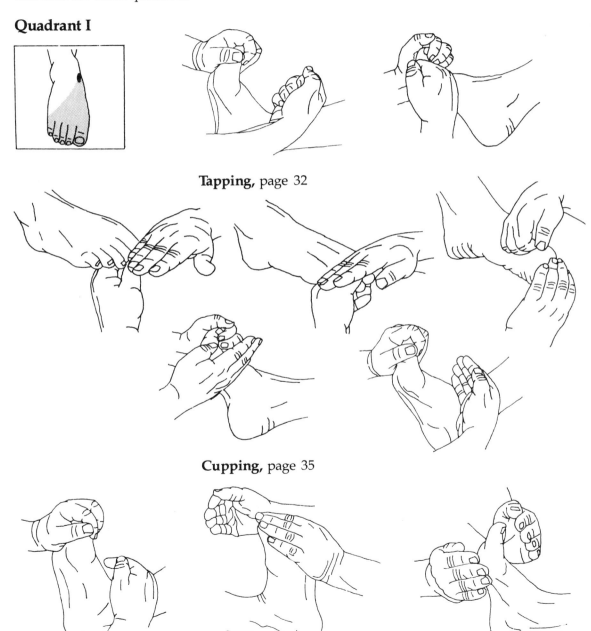

Tapping, page 32

Cupping, page 35

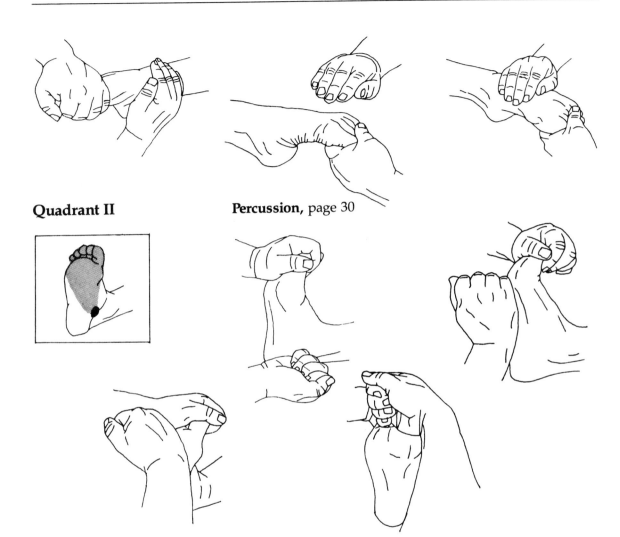

Quadrant II

Percussion, page 30

Tapping, page 32

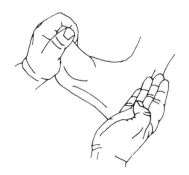

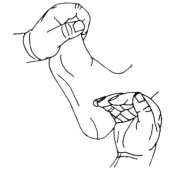

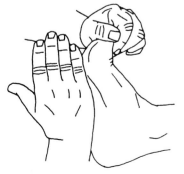

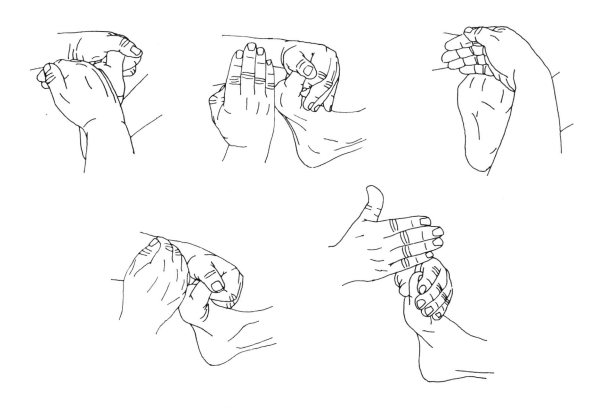

Cupping, page 35

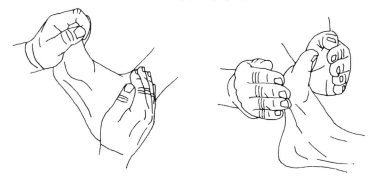

Quadrant III

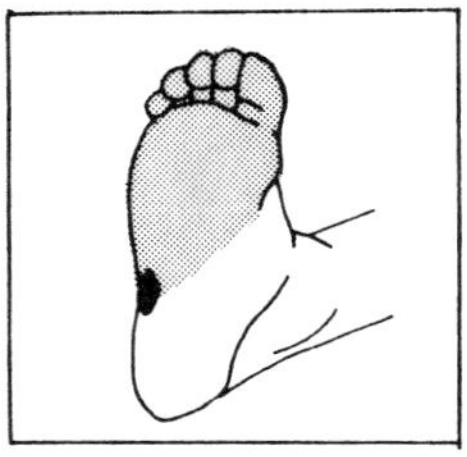

Percussion, page 30

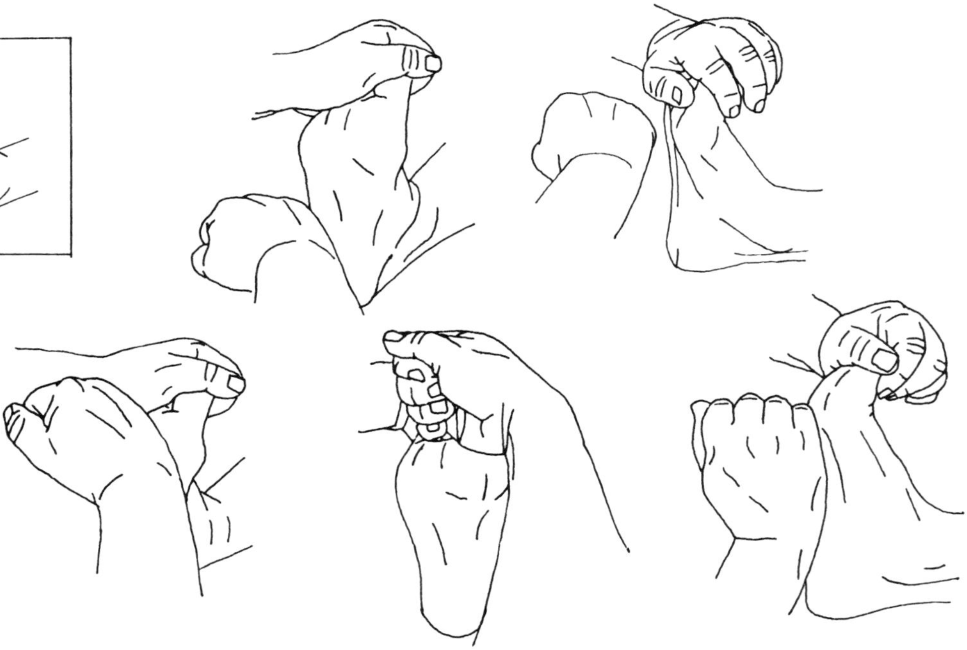

Tapping, page 32

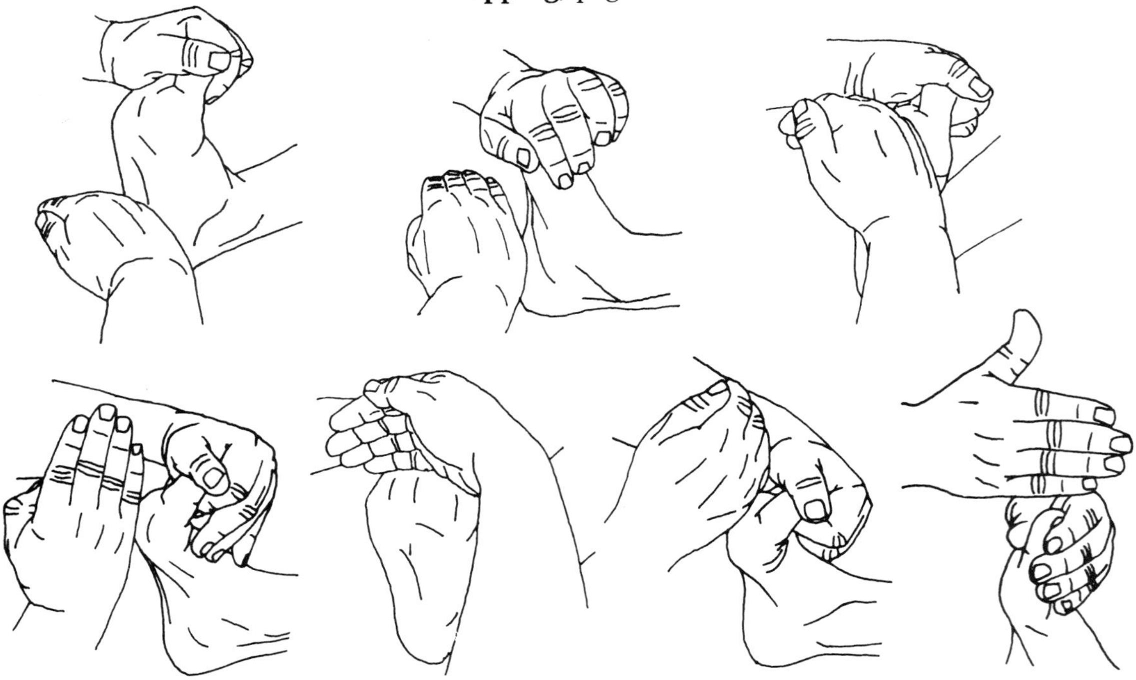

Cupping, page 35

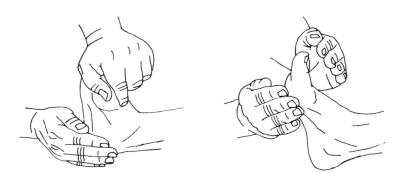

Feathering, See Kunz and Kunz, *The Complete Guide to Foot Reflexology,* Prentice-Hall, Inc., 1982.

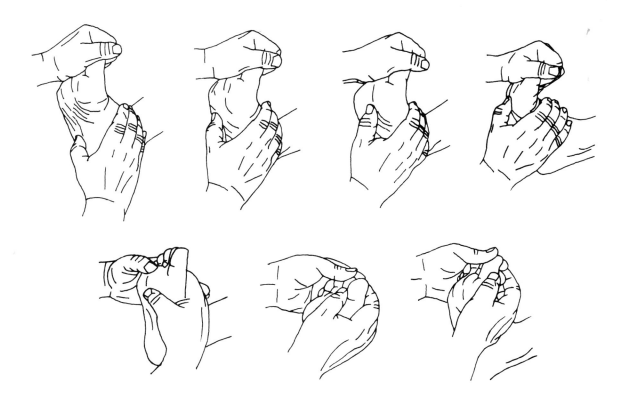

Quadrant IV

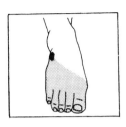

Tapping, page 32

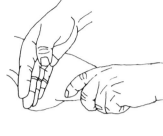

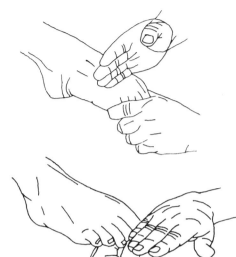

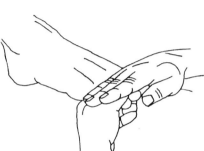

Cupping, page 35

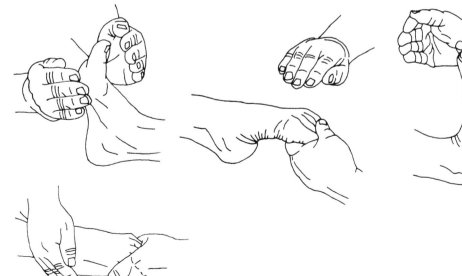

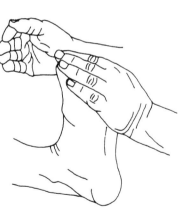

THE ANKLE

The four major muscle groups of the foot pass through the ankle. Their close proximity in the ankle creates areas of interest for the application of stride replication® techniques.

Tapping, page 32

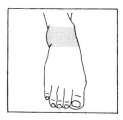

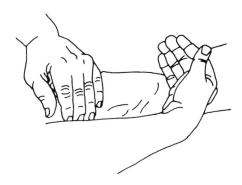

Percussion, page 30

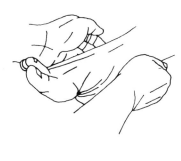

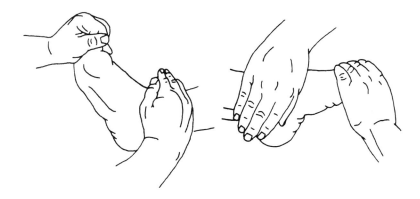

Special Interests: Propriocise®

Special Interests: Propriocise®   links technique and movement practiced. See also Circling, page 52 .

Integrated movement is noted by a symbol indicating which quadrants the foot is moved through during the application of technique.

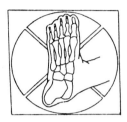

Movement at a joint is noted by a bone chart.

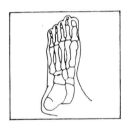

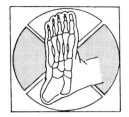

Side to side mover, page 50

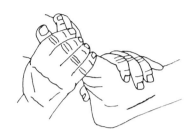
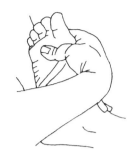

Side to side, page 45

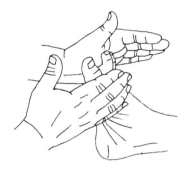
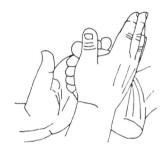

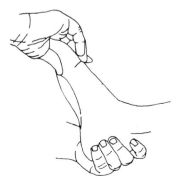

Foot flicking, page 48

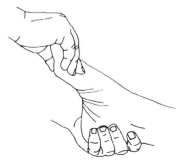

Foot flicking (toe), page 48

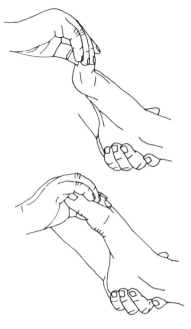
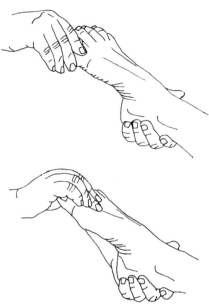

Metatarsal fan, page 44

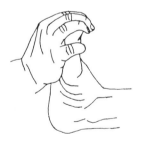
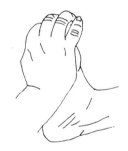
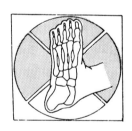

Metatarsal fan, page 44

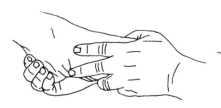
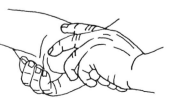
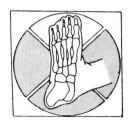

Plantar rocker, page 47

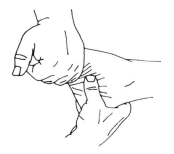 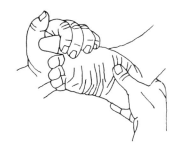

Heel to toe mover, page 46

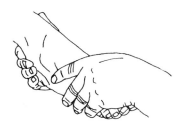 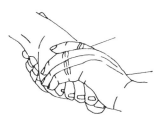

Heel to toe mover, page 46

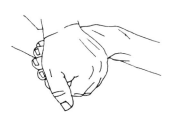 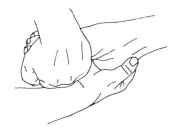

Side to side, page 45

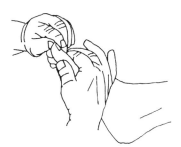 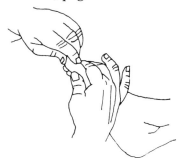 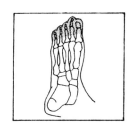

Pull, page 51

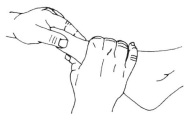 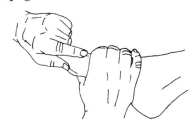

Metatarsal grasp, page 50

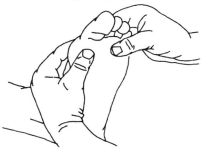 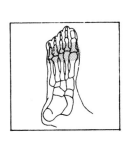

Metatarsal lever, page 49

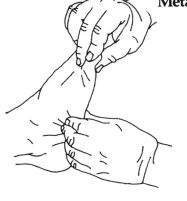 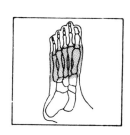

You, The Practitioner

The translation of a belief system into a profession requires a perception of professional practice and the discipline to practice within the defined boundaries. The boundaries are defined partially by the profession and partially by society.

The evolution of reflexology from a verbal tradition to a profession follows a path common to emerging professions. To recognize a profession, society first must be assured of the good intentions, definition, service provided, and mastery of the craft. These identifiable elements provide a focus for reflexology as an emerging profession.

The Kunz Method of Reflexology has been recognized as a form of complementary medicine by The Institute for Complementary Medicine in England. (See "Postscript," page 140).This formal recognition of Kunz Method was made possible by the anticipation of questions to be answered by an emerging profesion. The Kunz Method was accepted as a credible practice for its ethical, professional, and scientific basis. It is possible for a profession to shape its image.

IMAGE OF A PROFESSION

The image of a profession is created by society's perception of it. Because reflexology has a fundamentally different approach to the body than the medical model, its professional image has yet to be established. Its theoretical basis is a matter of debate within the profession itself. Society's current demand is that the profession define itself within scientific boundaries.

The demand for definition is required by a society that wants to purchase a service yet be protected from charlatans who would separate its members from their money for no benefit. Thus have evolved the Fair Practice Acts which require that the consumer be fully and fairly apprised of the service that is to be purchased.

Society has seen it necessary to define health practitioners in particular because of the "sacred trust" implied in dealing with the most intimate part of a person, his or her body. The claim of reflexology to physically affect the body must be met by an accountability to explain the serive offered and the benefit gained. Without this — a valued commodity to be gained — a profession is not granted sanction by the community to practice on a formal level. Anecdotal medicine that cites observation without causal relationship based on scientific literature has little chance of its physical claims being taken seriously on a formal level.

Furthermore, a professional's image is conveyed by the code of ethics, values, norms, and symbols of his or her profession. Thus, when the individual consumer seeks the services of an individual practitioner, the consumer is assured that the profession has guidelines that it deems necessary to ask its professionals to follow.

The challenge to any profession is to meet the public's needs and expectations. These are signaled by laws, the marketplace response, and acceptance of the profession in general. At this time, the practitioner defines his or her practice and standards without the support and definition of an established profession.

The discussion that follows reflects the growth of a profession within boundaries chosen to balance the goals of the profession and its perception by society.

PRACTICES OF A PROFESSION

Reflexology is:
1. the physical act of
2. applying pressure to the feet
3. with specific thumb, finger and hand techniques
4. which do not use oil or lotion
5. based on a system of zones and areas reiterating an image of the body on the feet.
6. with a premise that such work effects a physical change in the body.

Society, for its part, has seen it necessary to ask for further clarification of the professional application of techniques based on this premise. The request for clarification is a request for an identity for reflexology; for (1) scientific validity, (2) assurance that licensed professions are protected, and (3) assurance that the consumer is fairly informed of the service. Accuracy and fairness are the key words here. With the exchange of money, the services promised should be provided. (Fair Trade Acts with this emphasis are in effect in many states.) It is the responsibility of the professional practitioner to fairly inform the consumer of services promised. Thus, it becomes a part of the professional's practice to clearly label to the consumer the service that is offered.

Keeping these generalities in mind, boundaries can be set that afford the practitioner the opportunity to infuse his or her work with individual creative expression and meet the ethical and legal concerns of society.

The following discussion is not intended as legal counsel. Should you require legal services, we suggest that you consult your attorney. Laws vary from state to state and municipality to municipality. Different concerns have arisen in different areas. For example, antiprostitution laws in certain municipalities require a massage license, special zoning, and/or the wearing of a white lab coat to professionally work with another's body if the practitioner is not a member of an exempted profession (e.g., doctor, nurse, dentist).

LABELING Describing the service offered begins with the labels used for the service. For example, foot massage is not reflexology, and reflexology is not foot massage. In the first instance, oils, lotions, or creams are used in foot massage, but in reflexology the basic commodity is techniques applied to a bare foot. In the second instance, massage is a licensed profession in many areas, and the use of the term *foot massage* gives the impression that the practitioner meets standards of massage licensure.

VOCABULARY Foot reflexology has an established reputation and tradition. Use of terms such as therapy, physical therapy, cure, heal, doctor, reverend, treatment, and patient should be carefully considered as professional vocabulary words. Their use can be misconstrued as the practice of another profession.

CREDENTIALS Further description of a professional is gained through presentation of credentials. Honesty is the best policy. The profession of reflexology has yet to establish an accreditation process that is universally accepted. There is no accepted training time within which the professional learns his or her craft. As in many fields, however, experience is a substitute for lack of credentialed training. Thus, the reflexologist who has fourteen hours of training and fourteen years of experience is recognized for his or her experience.

MIXING MODALITIES Reflexology is not a coverall for any and all services. The consumer has a right to know the qualifications of the practitioner, including other professional credentials. This assures the consumer that the practitioner is licensed to practice any additional modalities that he or she might offer the consumer.

Mixing modalities presents multiple considerations. What labels are the services offered under? When the reflexologist offers shiatsu and herbs as part of reflexology work, what job title should he or she be given? Can the ethical considerations of finding a problem by reflexology and then selling another product or service as a solution be surmounted?

Will the additional products and services interfere with the service of reflexology that the practitioner is committed to providing the client? At the time an initial contact is made with a client, should the client be informed that the practitioner offers services in addition to reflexology?

Further ramifications of mixing modalities include the potential misrepresentation of the foot reflexology chart on the wall of a professional's office, especially one without a disclaimer. (See below).   It is the combination of a foot reflexology chart and any other product or service which may be construed by the law as a combination of diagnostic and prescriptive procedures. This may be construed as practicing medicine without a license.

DISCLAIMERS

Display of a foot or hand reflexology chart in the work place should include a disclaimer that is readable by the client. Thus, the practitioner is seen to be responsible in informing the client of the nature of his or her services.

> **Reflexology is not intended to be a substitute for medical care. If you have a health problem, consult a medical professional. This chart represents the "reiteration theory" of the body, a fundamental concept in reflexology. It is not intended to be applied as a diagnostic tool.**

Further consideration should be given to any material in the work place that can be read or handled by the client. Any material that contains testimonials without a disclaimer and any material that does not direct the client to medical care should he or she have a medical problem belongs in the practitioner's private library.

Disclaimers also are used to demonstrate that the practitioner is responsibly clarifying the nature of his or her services for the consumer. A written disclaimer, signed by the client and displayed in the work place, clearly defines the practitioner's role.

DO NOT PRACTICE A LICENSED PROFESSION

Practices such as medical care, massage, chiropractics, and podiatry (i.e., nail trimming) are services licensed to a specific group by the state to protect the public. The practice of such a profession without a license is a violation of the law.

TEACHING

Responsibilities are assumed by teachers or institutions that offer certificates or diplomas. It should be made clear to the student that the certificate does not provide legal sanction to practice reflexology or any other profession.

THE ROLE OF THE PRACTITIONER AS AN ADVOCATE OF SELF-HELP

Self-help is the involvement of the client in his or her own program of wellness. Reflexology, stride replication® , and propriocise® provide techniques that are opportunities to practice and exercise the hand's capabilities. As in any exercise program, time spent exercising the foot is a factor in the program. The addition of the client's self-help program is an opportunity to spend more time exercising. (See *Hand and Foot Reflexology, A Self-Help Guide,* Kevin and Barbara Kunz, Prentice-Hall, Inc., 1984.)

DO NOT WORK ON AN UNDIAGNOSED PROBLEM

An undiagnosed problem that is acute enough to cause the client concern but which has not yet been examined by a physician should not be worked. For example, a painful toe may be an injured toe that needs medical care. When in doubt, refer the client to medical personnel.

RESPECT AN INDIVIDUAL'S TOLERANCE TO PAIN

Pain is not an activity that needs to be practiced. There is a difference between a client's comment of, "It hurts good" and one of "It hurts." One method of eliciting comments on the amount of pressure preferred by the client is to ask, "Will you tell me if the pressure is too much?" This is especially appropriate when applying techniques to areas you think might be sensitive.

THE FUTURE OF A PROFESSION

Society has its reasons for requesting that the profession of reflexology identify itself within appropriate boundaries. The discipline itself has the ultimate responsibility to establish boundaries for its practitioners. The continued growth of the profession is possible, but only with the agreement of its members for the need to reconcile its practices with the needs of society.

What service is provided by reflexology?
The central issue is in the interpretation of the definition of reflexology. If a basic premise of reflexology is that work on feet affects a physical change in the body, what is the nature of that change? Words become important at this point in the discussion.

The observed effect of reflexology is described in traditional reflexology as:
- relaxation of tension
- normalization of gland and organ function
- improvement of blood and nerve circulation

Eastern philosophies such as acupuncture are allowed by Western society to explain their workings in terms of mysticism. Western philosophies such as reflexology are not allowed such mysticism. In the Western culture, it is seen as important to attach a cause to an effect. Reflexology had only work on feet as a cause to mysteriously explain its effects. To those who have observed the effects, the effects are reason enough to believe. To be recognized as a profession in Western society, however, scientific cause must be assigned to the effect noted.

Reflexology's explanations included: no explanation at all, an energy system without a known physiological structure similar to acupuncture, and others. Current science recognizes physical explanations for physical effects.

Words are important. The observed effects of reflexology do, however, have an explanation in physical terms. Any sensory input causes a change in the body's operating tempo. Reflexology, stride replication®, and propriocise® techniques are practices of pressure, stretch, and movement. These sensations link the foot to the rest of the body.

What service is provided by reflexology?

The service provided by reflexology is the application of pressure, stretch, and movement techniques resulting in relaxation, body awareness, and locomotive energy savings. This interpretation of reflexology, the belief system, to reflexology, the science, is a matter of words. A further examination of relaxation of tension, normalization of gland and organ function, and improvement of blood and nerve circulation provides a link between reflexology and the premises necessary to be accepted by society as a valued profession.

What kind of assessment can be made with reflexology?

Assessment and evaluation in reflexology are a reflection of the body whole. While the vocabulary of assessment in reflexology is based on body parts, such as kidney or liver, such assessment has the potential for being misconstrued as the making of a diagnosis or the practice of medicine without a license. Do not diagnose, prescribe, or treat for a specific illness.

Assessment is necessary to proceed in any endeavor. In addition to the application of pressure, stretch, and movement techniques, the practitioner provides an assessment that both practitioner and client understand to be in the language of reflexology and not of medical practice.

In reflexology, assessment is made by observation (primarily, of what the thumb feels). Observation is categorized, as, for example, a kidney reiterative area. By using terms such as "kidney reiterative area," the practitioner further emphasizes his or her awareness of the service offered by reflexology.

Reflexology is the practice of sensory signals, the exercise of the foot's potential. Such practice is based on certain causal relationships. These causal relationships are not the same as those used by the traditional medical community in the diagnosis of a medical problem.

The sensory assessment garnered by the reflexologist is a reflection of the body whole and the demands made upon it. The demands are those of walking upright and acting in relation to gravity. The goal in the application of technique is the exercise of the sensors that make weight-carrying and manipulation possible. The important assessment is the one made by the body as a sensory technique is applied. A picture is provided to the body from which judgments are made. Judgments are in the body's language of muscle tension, among others.

Is it necessary to license reflexology?

Ultimately, it probably will be necessary for the profession of reflexology to comply with the professional codes in effect in many states and countries. Within a professional code, the profession is given definition and boundaries.

The basis of licensure is the regulation of a profession by the state government for the protection of public health, safety, and welfare. Licensure varies from profession to profession with the amount of responsibility assumed by the practitioner. The beauty operator, for example, assumes less liability than the brain surgeon.

As an emerging profession, the perception reflexologists have of reflexology will be a determiner in any discussion of the licensure of the profession. The closer the perception is to health care as the service provided, the greater the requirement for increasing responsibility by the professional, as well as increasingly higher standards of education and training. Thus, the definition within which reflexology is considered for licensure determines where in the framework of professions it will be placed.

What is the future of accreditation in reflexology?

There is no certification required to practice reflexology professionally. There is a real need for the professional reflexologist to have credentials. A universally recognized certificate of qualification should be a part of any profession. There is no certification process which we recognize as valid at this time. The educational material, length of training time, and testing procedures do not currently exist to serve as a basis for valid certification.

A profession exists by staying within the laws. A profession grows by seeking the highest standards of practice. Accreditation is an indicator of that search. The matter to be discussed by the profession as a whole is the manner in which its credentials process can be described and given validity by the public and other professionals. The responsibility is for each method of reflexology to define itself and its certification process to create an informed consumer and a protected practitioner.

What should a reflexologist say to a client?

Client: "I looked at a reflexology chart and it said that the sore area on my foot is related to the kidneys. Is there something wrong with my kidneys?"

Reflexologist: "Reflexology charts represent the reiteration theory. This is a theory of how the body communicates with itself. It is in no way indicative of ill health nor is it a diagnostic tool."

Client: "I don't know what's wrong with my foot but it hurts. Can you work on it and help it?"

Reflexologist: "No, if you have an undiagnosed foot problem, we suggest that you consult a podiatrist or an orthopedic surgeon."

Client: "Can you help me with my back problem?"

Reflexologist: "No, I provide no medical services. I suggest that you see a medical professional."

Client: "But I've been to all the doctors and they haven't helped."

Reflexologist: "What you are asking is whether or not I can treat you for a specific illness. By state law, only a doctor may provide such a service. I am not an alternative to medical care."

Client: "Can you recommend a vitamin to help my condition?"

Reflexologist: "No, I cannot. An answer to your question is construed as prescribing or practicing medicine without a license."

Client: "The doctor gave me this medicine but I'm not sure about taking it. What do you think?"

Reflexologist: "If you have questions about your medication, I suggest that you consult your doctor."

Client: "What can reflexology do for me?"

Reflexologist: "Reflexology works with the communication system of the body. A reflexologist provides sensory experience to a neglected sensory organ, the feet. Our theory is that improved communication improves the organization of the body and develops a sense of bodily awareness, just as the study of wine appreciation helps develop the body's sense of taste."

Postscript

POSTSCRIPT

The Kunz Method of Reflexology is designed to meet needs to define a practice of reflexology within ethical, scientific, and legal boundaries. Recognition of this approach has been achieved by the acceptance of the Kunz Method as a form of complementary medicine by the Institute for Complementary Medicine in England. The Kunz Method joins chiropractics, osteopathy, acupuncture, herbal medicine, and homeopathy as a "style of medical practice that regards health and disease in the terms of the whole person." (I.C.M. literature) The Kunz Method was selected for its ethical, professional, and scientific basis as well as the clinical and instructional work of Robert Dallamore, our British representative.

The written work of the Kunz Method is on file as the literature of the field in England. That literature is:

Kunz and Kunz, *The Complete Guide to Foot Reflexology*, Prentice-Hall, Inc., 1982

Kunz and Kunz, *Hand and Foot Reflexology, A Self-Help Guide*, Prentice-Hall, Inc., 1984

Kunz and Kunz, *Hand Reflexology Workbook*, Prentice-Hall, Inc. 1985

Kunz and Kunz, *The Practitioner's Guide to Reflexology*, Prentice-Hall, Inc., 1985

Kunz and Kunz, *Reflexions*, Reflexology Research Project, Volume 1, Number 1 (July 1980) through Volume 6, Number 1 (Jan./Feb./Mar., 1985).

We will continue to document practices of the Kunz Method to further notify the practitioner and the public of our intent to strive for a quality practice, responsive to the needs of the community served. In addition, we hope to plant the seeds for future research, literature, and study among reflexologists.

Appendix

DIRECTORY ANNOUNCEMENT
and PARTICIPATION by POLL

The poll results that follow are a prelude to an international directory of reflexologists, that will reflect the perceptions of those who practice the craft. The poll was conducted by sociologist Jill Schneider. Over one hundred fifty individuals responded.

GOALS OF THE DIRECTORY:

Facilitate communication among those interested in or practicing reflexology.

Give the public information about reflexology and reflexologists.

Signal the desire by the profession of reflexology to act in fair regard to the consumer and to self-regulate the practices of the profession.

GOALS OF THE POLL:

Design a directory that accurately reflects the opinions of those who practice reflexology.

Enable each reflexologist to participate in this process.

Define and describe the various styles and practices of reflexology.

Question		Response		No.	%
1.	How long have you been a reflexologist?	1.	0- 1 years	33	25
			1- 5 years	64	48
			5-10 years	20	15
			10-15 years	9	7
			15-40 years	7	5
2.	Why did you become a reflexologist?	2.			
	a. To pursue a personal health problem		a. 50		
	b. Because a member of my family had a health problem		b. 37		
	c. Because I wanted to help people		c. 112		
	d. Because I wanted to make money		d. 19		
	e. Looking for a profession or a job		e. 45		
	f. Other (specify)		f. 7		

3. How did you learn reflexology?
    a. Self taught
    b. From a book
    c. From an individual
    d. From a class

3.   a.   37
      b.   62
      c.   45
      d. 109

4. I am _____ years old.

4. **Age Sheet Summary**
    (1) oldest - 82
    (2) youngest - 24
    (3) most frequent age - 43
    (4) Average age of 140 - 46.8

5. My profession is _____

5. **31—reflexologist**
    34—allied profession (other body/health work)
    12—traditional medical profession
    43—other professions
    19—retired, housewife, student

6. I live in (city, state, province, country)

6. **Thirty-two states in the United States and eleven foreign countries were listed in response to the question.**

7. Do you get paid to do reflexology on other people's feet?

7.
	No.	%
yes	85	64
no	22	16
sometimes	26	20

8. I am ____male ____female

8.
	No.	%
male	67	46
female	79	54

9. **I have the following education:**
    a. Completed grade school through ninth grade
    b. Have high school diploma
    c. Have _____ years of college
    d. Have special training such as nursing, technical skills, apprentice programs, etc. (explain)

9.   a.   8
      b. 37
      c. 97
      d. 36

10. Who do you usually work on?
    a. Myself
    b. My family
    c. Friends
    d. People who request my services.

10.   a.   58
      b.   77
      c   70
      d. 123

11. The people I practice reflexology on are usually:
    a. Younger than me.
    b. Older than me.
    c. Of all ages.

11.   **a. 6**
             b. 10
             c. 132

12. The people I usually work on are:
    a. Chronically ill, i.e. have arthritis, diabetes, heart disease, cancer, or other long term, ongoing health problem.
    b. Have a minor problem like sinuses or a back ache.
    c. Temporarily sick: have a cold, the flu or are recovering from an unusual health problem like an operation.
    d. Are not ill, but get their feet worked on because they see it as a way to stay healthy or reduce stress.
    e. Are not ill, but just like the way reflexology feels.

12.   **a. 87**

             b. 99

             c. 67

             d. 88

             e. 50

13. The people I like to work on the most are: (describe your favorite clients in a few words)

13. **53—open minded**
     19—believers
     11—seeking alternatives
     35—(specific disorder listed)
      2—women with small feet
      1—those who wash feet
     25—miscellaneous others

14. The people I think would benefit the most from reflexology are:

14. **58—anyone**
     20—open minded
     15—stress
     12—seniors
     10—chronically ill
      8—healthy people
     15—miscellaneous others

15. Do you get to work on these people?
    yes _____ no _____

15.

	No.	**%**
yes	**108**	**91**
no	**11**	**9**

16. I think people I practice on come to me because:
    a. They think reflexology helps them along with traditional medicine.
    b. They don't think traditional medicine can do what reflexology does.
    c. They have lost faith in their doctors.

16.   **a. 83**

             b. 59
             c. 61

17.	I think there are areas on the feet that correspond to areas on the body. Agree Disagree	17.		**No.**	**%**
			Agree	143	100
			Disagree	0	0

18.	I think reflexology stimulates a flow of blood to particular places in the body Agree Disagree	18.	**Agree**	133	96
			Disagree	5	4

19.	I think that reflexology affects calcium deposits in the body. Agree Disagree	19.	**Agree**	123	90
			Disagree	14	10

20.	I think people get sick when they are unhappy or under stress. Agree Disagree	20.	**Agree**	144	99
			Disagree	1	.7

21.	I think Mildred Carter has the correct approach to foot reflexology. Agree Disagree Don't Know	21.	**Agree**	50	38
			Disagree	27	20
			Don't know	55	42

22.	I think there are zones dividing the body and reflexology works through these zones. Agree Disagree Don't Know	22.	**Agree**	127	91
			Disagree	1	.7
			Don't know	13	9

23.	I don't know how reflexology really works but I think it is a valid way to help health problems. Agree Disagree	23.	**Agree**	121	92
			Disagree	10	8

24.	I think the scientists and doctors could figure out reflexology if they tried. Agree Disagree	24.	**Agree**	114	90
			Disagree	12	10

25.	I think the reflexologist benefits from working on people as much as the people being worked on benefit. Agree Disagree	25.	**Agree**	120	88
			Disagree	17	12

26.	When I am sick/upset I can't do as good a job on a client as when I am calm/healthy. Agree Disagree	26.	**Agree**	131	94
			Disagree	8	6

27.	I think physical contact with another person can help many health problems. Agree Disagree	27.	**Agree**	140	100
			Disagree	0	0

28.	I think your mind and body are connected and one affects the other when it comes to health; a strong mind in a healthy body. Agree Disagree	28.	**Agree**	139	99
			Disagree	2	1

29.	I think you can get instant results with reflexology. Yes No Sometimes	29.	**Yes**	30	21
			no	7	5
			Sometimes	107	74

30.	I think reflexology has a cumulative effect; you have to do it for several weeks or months before you get results. Agree Disagree Both	30.	**Agree**	29	22
			Disagree	14	10
			Both	92	68

			No.	%
31. Sometimes reflexology can't do any good. Agree Disagree	31.	Agree Disagree	63 67	48 52
32. Reflexology could replace doctors. Agree Disagree	32.	Agree Disagree	9 127	7 93
33. How much do you charge for your services? (U.S. dollars) a. under $10.00 b. $11.00 to $20.00 c. $21.00 to $30.00 d. $31.00 or more e. People pay me whatever they want. f. I accept donations.	33.	a. b. c. d. e. f.	20 62 11 5 24	23 47 8 4 18
34. How would you describe yourself? a. Part-time professional reflexologist b. Part-time professional reflexologist working towrds full time c. Full time professional reflexologist d. Not professional, just practicing reflexologist.	34.	a. b. c. d.	28 35 34 40	20 26 25 29
35. Where do you work? (Check more than one if necessary) a. Home b. Office c. Home of client d. Other professional's office	35.	a. b. c. d.	79 46 4 6	60 34 2 4
36. How do you attract new clientele? a. Word of mouth b. Advertising c. Demonstrations d. Other	36.	a. b. c. d.	120 43 50	
37. How many pairs of feet do you work on per week? (If you work on a person twice a week, count him or her twice.)	37.	0- 5 pairs 5-10 pairs 10-15 pairs 15-20 pairs 21-50 pairs	39 36 20 22 17	29 27 15 17 12
38. How long do you work on a pair of feet in general?	38.	0-15 min. 15-30 min. 30-45 min. 45-60 min. Over 60	5 28 62 38 4	4 20 45 28 3

39.	In what position are you when working feet? a. Seated directly facing the individual b. Standing c. Other	**39.**	a. b.	130 15	

40.	How would you describe reflexology as a profession (Check yes or no in response to statement) YesNo	**40.**		Yes	No
	Personally rewarding			130	1
	Provides adequate financial remuneration			56	45
	Professionally rewarding (provides adequate recognition from public and other professions)			52	48

41.	Do you, or have you, worked professionally with other health professionals? (e.g. M.D., podiatrist, osteopath, chiropractor)	**41.**	Independent . . . . 63% Chiropractor . . . . 16% Physician . . . . 13% Other health professionals 8%

42.	What service or services do you provide to your clientele with your reflexology work? a. Working with reflex areas b. Working to eliminate calcium deposits c. Relaxation d. Health care for a problem e. Sensory experience	**42.**	a. b. c. d. e.	No. 116 77 112 76 43

43.	Have you had legal difficulty in practicing reflexology?YesNo	**43.**	Yes No	4 126

44.	Do you know of others who have? YesNo	**44.**	Yes No	7 110

45.	Do you sell products as a part of your business? YesNo a. foot reflexology products b. corrective foot devices c. herbs d. vitamins e. exercise equipment f. other	**45.**	Yes No a. b. c. d. e. f.	7 110 14 8 20 23 15 19

46.	Do you provide services other than reflexology? YesNo a. massage b. other body work c. nail clipping d. counseling e. spiritual advice f. other	**46.**	Yes No a. b. c. d. e. f.	85 48 52 38 10 36 30 28

47. For what reason(s) do you sell other products or services?
    a. Provide the client with needed service
    b. Income opportunity
    c. Other

47.   a.   39
       b.   16

Note: Of the 85 respondants who provide other services, 45 are licensed to do so, have education required to provide service (e.g. counseling), or have a waiver of licensure because of trained profession (e.g. beauticians and nurses are exempted from massage acts). Some of the other respondants are not required to be licensed to offer the other service, some provide services at no expense (e.g. counseling, spiritual advice), and some do not charge for reflexology and/or the other service.

Written responses to Question 2.

"I love working on feet." "The results were so dramatic I continued the sessions and I am learning this so I can help my reflexologist when she isn't feeling well." "Enjoyed working on feet, too." " Had results in myself from it." "I received so much help myself — wanted to help others." "Because feet are so nice." "I've been told by many that I have high sensitivity and good energy in my hands, and reflexology is an ideal medium for this natural gift." "To give people a choice in health care." "To supplement my work as a physical therapist, to use as another healing modality." "I believe in the holistic approach in eliminating illnesses." "Interested in holistic health." "Personal health and the health of my children." "Looking for a satisfying and rewarding career." "Because I relieved myself of prostate gland trouble." "Interested in health problems." "It is the most wonderful thing I have ever encountered." "It would be another occupation to help when I leave present job." "It works beautifully." "To help people in a natural way with their health." "After retirement, I needed something to do — not to become a recluse." "The whole concept fascinated me and I had to learn it." "Advice of several older people who had benefited from reflexology." "To help people." "To advance my own life." "I really enjoy it, as well as helping people." "To complement my career as a massage therapist." "Upgrading skills." "A long time interest and commitment to holistic healing." "Sounded interesting, and I felt there was validity to the practice." "Because I could bring comfort and relief to others." "I was gifted with touch for points — wanted to apply it and satisfy people, and self." "Because I wanted to help my family maintain its health." "To make people feel better." "I felt I had the 'touch' and ability." "To take greater responsibility for the health care of myself and my family." "I'm a borderline diabetic and wanted to get myself off medication. I've been off it for a year and I'm doing great." "It started as a hobby." "To complement my other disciplines." "I wanted to help my fellow men to better health." "Reflexology is an excellent alternative method." "To augment my profession as a Chiropodist." "Because I was led into it." "To have a healthy body." "To be a professional at a health center." "It fascinated me." "Fascinated by procedure and results." "Interesting and it works." "I believe in it." "Could not afford nor wanted doctors and hospitals — and belief that God helps those who help themselves." "Interest in helping myself and others." "As an adjunct to my other therapy practice." "To also explore every avenue available for increasing my awareness of how my body works and to help my body do its job of rejuvenation naturally." "As part of wholistic natural healing." "As a means to improved health to use with family and friends."

FOOT REFLEXOLOGY CHARTS

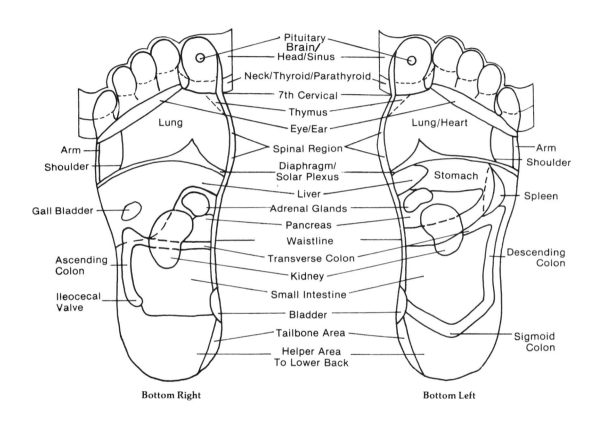

Pituitary
Brain/
Head/Sinus
Neck/Thyroid/Parathyroid
7th Cervical
Thymus
Lung
Eye/Ear
Lung/Heart
Arm
Shoulder
Arm
Spinal Region
Shoulder
Diaphragm/
Solar Plexus
Stomach
Liver
Spleen
Gall Bladder
Adrenal Glands
Pancreas
Waistline
Descending
Colon
Ascending
Colon
Transverse Colon
Kidney
Ileocecal
Valve
Small Intestine
Bladder
Tailbone Area
Sigmoid
Colon
Helper Area
To Lower Back

Bottom Right
Bottom Left

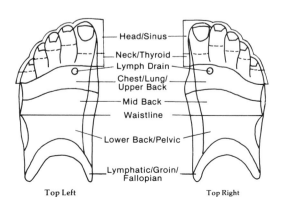

Head/Sinus
Neck/Thyroid
Lymph Drain
Chest/Lung/
Upper Back
Mid Back
Waistline
Lower Back/Pelvic
Lymphatic/Groin/
Fallopian

Top Left
Top Right

FOOT REFLEXOLOGY CHARTS

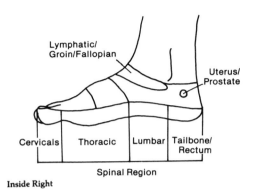

Lymphatic/
Groin/Fallopian

Uterus/
Prostate

Cervicals | Thoracic | Lumbar | Tailbone/
Rectum

Spinal Region

Inside Right

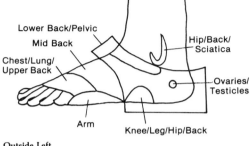

Lower Back/Pelvic

Mid Back

Chest/Lung/
Upper Back

Hip/Back/
Sciatica

Ovaries/
Testicles

Arm

Knee/Leg/Hip/Back

Outside Left

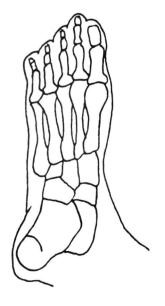

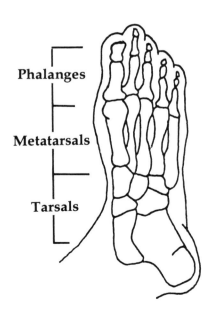

Phalanges

Metatarsals

Tarsals

BIBLIOGRAPHY

Bakan, David. *Is Phrenology Foolish?*, Readings in Experimental Psychology Today, Del Mar, CRM Books, 1967, PP. 3-9.

Cousins, Norman. *Anatomy of an Illness*, New York: W.W. Norton and Co., 1979.

Dale, Ralph Alan. "The Micro-Acupuncture Systems," *American Journal of Acupuncture*, Vol. 4, No. 1, March, and Vol. 4, No. 3, July-September, 1976, pp. 7-24, pp. 196-224.

Gellhorn, Ernst. *Principles of Autonomic Somatic Integration*, Minneapolis: University of Minnesota Press, 1967.

Gellhorn, Ernst, and G.W. Loofburrow. *Emotions and Emotional Disorders: A Neuro-Physiological Study*, New York: Harper and Row, 1963.

Guyton, Arthur C. *Basic Human Physiology: Normal Function and Mechanisms of Disease*, Philadelphia, W.B. Saunders Company, 1969.

Jung, Carl G. *Man and His Symbols*, New York, Dell Publishing Co., 1968.

Miller, Jonathan. *The Body in Question*, New York Random House, 1982.

Montagu, Ashley. *Touching: The Human Significance of the Skin*, New York: Harper and Row, 1971.

Napier, John. "The Antiquity of Human Walking," *Scientific American*, April 1967, pp. 48-48.

Napier, John. "The Evolution of the Hand," *Scientific American*, December, 1962, pp. 49-55.

Pribram, Karl H. *Languages of the Brain: Experimental Paradoxes and Principles of Neuropsychology*, Englewood Cliffs, NJ: Prentice-Hall, Inc., 1971.

Schneider, Jill. "A Definition of a Profession and Some Notes Pertaining to Reflexology," 1982.

Selye, Hans. *Stress Without Distress*, New York, The New American Library, Inc., 1974.

Simonton, O. Carl, Matthews-Simonton, Stephanie, and Creighton, James L. *Getting Well Again*, New York, Bantam Books, 1978.

Staff, Board of Medical Quality Assurance, State of California, "Proposal for Revision of Section 2052 of the Medical Practices Act," 1982.

Thompson, Richard F. *Foundation of Physiological Psychology,* New York: Harper and Row, 1967.

INDEX

acupuncture, 4, 10-11, 135
adaptation, 13-14, 16
ankle, 64
archestructure, 4
archetype, 3

body awareness, 13, 21

Complete Guide to Foot Reflexology, the, 17, 24
continuing relationship, 62

directional movement, 15, 18, 19, 59
   dorsiflexion, 15, 18, 19, 41
   eversion, 15, 18, 19, 39
   inversion, 15, 18, 19, 38
   plantarflexion, 15, 18, 19, 40
disclaimer, 133

endorphin, 10
energy, 13
evaluation, 27, 54
exercise, 20, 21

fight or flight, 9
Fitzgerald, William, 3
flexibility, 21, 22, 66
foot, 6-12
foot massage, 132
footstep, 14-15, 17, 18, 26
foot work, 2, 3, 21

Hand and Foot Reflexology, A Self-Help Guide, 134
Hand Reflexology Workbook, 17, 24
heel strike, 8, 14
Hirata, Dr., 3
holding hand, 24, 37, 43

Institute for Complementary Medicine, The, 130, 139
integrated movement, 65

Jung, Carl J., 3

Kunz Method of Reflexology, 130, 139

labeling, 132
licensing, 136
locomotion, 4, 8, 13

meridians, 4
movement, 2, 6, 21

neighboring relationship, 62, 65

observations, 54
   locomotive, 58-64, 94
   movement, 65-66, 99
   visual and touch, 55-57, 66
opposites, relationship of, 62, 65

pictograph, 5
pressure, 7, 11
proprioception, 7
propriocise® (definition of), 16, 17, 21

quadrant, 18, 58-59, 61
quadrant system, 18

referral relationships, 57, 90
reflexology (definition of), 16, 17
reiterative relationship, 11, 57, 90
relaxation, 20, 21

Schneider, Jill, 5
self-help, 134
Selye, Hans, 13
   General Adaptive Syndrome, 13
sensors, 7, 14
sensory organ, 6, 16
sensory signal, 17
   cupping, 35-37
   percussion, 30-32
   tapping, 32-34
shock absorption, 7, 10, 20, 26
shoes, 20
standing pattern, 16
stress, 3-16
stretch, 7, 26
stride, 7
stride mechanism, 8
stride path, 14, 16

stride replication® (definition of), 16, 17, 18
survival mechanism, 9, 11

terrain seeking, 20, 26

Wolff's Law, 10
working hand, 24, 26-27, 29, 43

zonal relationship, 57, 90
zones, 4

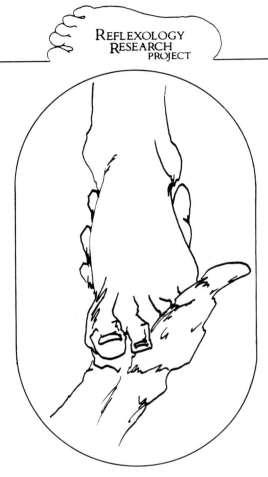

REFLEXOLOGY
RESEARCH
PROJECT

_____Yes, I would like to receive information about the Kunz Method of Reflexology.

_____Yes, I would like to receive information about a listing in the International
Directory of Reflexology.

Name _____

Address _____

City, State, Zip _____

Please mail completed form to:
Kunz Method of Reflexology
P.O. Box 35820, Stn. D, Albuquerque, New Mexico 87176